The Occupational Therapy Handbook:
Practice Education

Other books from M&K include:

Working with Children who need Long-term Respiratory Support
ISBN: 9781905539697

Research Issues in Health and Social Care
ISBN: 9781905395208

Timely Discharge from Hospital
ISBN: 9781905395550

Valuing People with a Learning Disability
ISBN: 9781905395666

A Pre-Reader for the Foundation Degree in Health and Social Care Practice
ISBN: 9781905539680

Preoperative Assessment & Perioperative Management
ISBN: 9781905539024

The Clinician's Guide to Chronic Disease Management for Long Term Conditions
ISBN: 9781905539154

The Occupational Therapy Handbook:

Practice Education

Tracey Polglase
Rachel Treseder

The Occupational Therapy Handbook: Practice Education
Tracey Polglase
Rachel Treseder

ISBN: 978-1-905539-75-8

First published 2012

British Library Cataloguing in Publication Data
A catalogue record for this book is available from the British Library

Notice
Clinical practice and medical knowledge constantly evolve. Standard safety precautions must be followed, but, as knowledge is broadened by research, changes in practice, treatment and drug therapy may become necessary or appropriate. Readers must check the most current product information provided by the manufacturer of each drug to be administered and verify the dosages and correct administration, as well as contraindications. It is the responsibility of the practitioner, utilising the experience and knowledge of the patient, to determine dosages and the best treatment for each individual patient. Any brands mentioned in this book are as examples only and are not endorsed by the publisher. Neither the publisher nor the authors assume any liability for any injury and/or damage to persons or property arising from this publication.

To contact M&K Publishing write to:
M&K Update Ltd · The Old Bakery · St. John's Street
Keswick · Cumbria CA12 5AS
Tel: 01768 773030 · Fax: 01768 781099
publishing@mkupdate.co.uk
www.mkupdate.co.uk

Designed and typeset by Mary Blood.
Printed in England by Ferguson Print, Keswick.

Contents

Tables

Figures

Preface

This book has been written as a current, specific occupational therapy text to reflect modern day occupational therapy practice and education. The editors were keen to create a current user-friendly textbook specifically in relation to Practice Education in Occupational Therapy, particularly in light of the developing role of occupational therapy in current practice. Many developments in practice education have re-focused the value that our profession places on occupation, particularly in role emerging placements and expanding areas of practice. These developments are captured in this text. The last text that addressed occupational therapy practice education in the UK was published in 1996, and is therefore rather dated. Other texts that have been produced have predominantly had a multi-professional focus and not addressed all the key occupational therapy issues in the depth required.

This book has been written specifically for occupational therapy students, newly qualified occupational therapists and educators. It is also a useful reference guide for academic tutors.

The book has been produced with specific discrete chapters, however where relevant cross referencing has been made explicit to direct the reader to other sections within the book.

Information has been presented in a variety of styles to allow the reader to quickly select specific elements or to explore a subject in depth. Tables, flow charts and figures have been used to summarise key issues.

At the end of the chapters there are reflective questions to assist the reader in applying the information to practice. There are also case studies in Chapter 5 – Assessment, Intervention and Evaluation sections to illustrate application of these elements. This is also reflective of the way students learn within higher education.

The book also looks to the future with a section focusing on where the profession is developing and current innovative practice.

It is hoped that those who read this book will find it informative and that it will encourage them to continue to develop their skills, whether they are students at the beginning of their career, newly qualified staff, educators (both inexperienced and experienced) or academic tutors. There is always something to learn, irrespective of your level of expertise. We have learnt a lot from writing this book and hope you also do when reading it!

Tracey and Rachel

About the Authors

Rachel Treseder
Occupational Therapy Lecturer at Cardiff University.
BSc (Hons) Occupational Therapy. MA Post Compulsory Education and Training.

Rachel has worked at Cardiff University as an Occupational Therapy Lecturer since 2004. She has a special interest in the development of occupational therapy into new and emerging areas, particularly within the voluntary sector. She also has experience of working as an occupational therapist in mental health and learning disabilities settings and more recently has developed a project working with young mothers from socially deprived backgrounds.

Tracey Polglase
Lead of the Practice Education Team in Wales and Lecturer at Cardiff University.
MSc Inter-professional Health Studies, Dip COT, PGCE (HE), PG Dip. Education Management, Registered OT.

Tracey has worked in education since 1998. She manages the Practice Education Team in Wales and lectures on the Occupational Therapy Programmes and on Post Graduate Inter-professional Modules within the School of Healthcare Studies. she has a particular interest in practice education, neurology, older adult rehabilitation and management. Prior to working in education She was Deputy Manager of an Occupational Therapy Service in Newport, Gwent. Tracey has also been instrumental in developing a Practice Education Database for use throughout Wales.

Carole Lawrie and **Maria Clarke** are Lecturers and Practice Education Co-ordinators at Cardiff University, Cardiff.

Liz Cade is a Lecturer and Practice Education Co-ordinator at Glyndwr University, Wrexham.

Part I

Theory and Context

Chapter 1
What is Practice Education?

Carole Lawrie and Tracey Polglase

Introduction

This chapter will define practice education and explore how it is incorporated into the curriculum. It will also discuss where practice education currently takes place and potential developments.

Practice placements are a 'highly important component of each course' (McClure, 2004 p. 7), preparing 'all health and social care professionals for academic award and registration to practice' (Turnock et al., 2005 p. 219). In occupational therapy education the World Federation of Occupational Therapy stipulates that the practical element must be a minimum of 1000 assessed hours (Hocking and Ness, 2002). Each university has a set number of placements that the student needs to successfully achieve. The number and length of placements may differ between the universities, but all need to meet the 1000 assessed hours.

Practice placements are undertaken in order to ensure that all students, at the end of their degree programme, are not only educationally well grounded in the theory of the profession but are also recognised as being competent, safe and fit to practise in order to be registered (Health Professions Council, 2005 (Health and Care Professions Council (HCPC) from 1 August 2012); Christiansen and Bell, 2010).

What is Practice Education in Occupational Therapy?

Occupational Therapy education is delivered as either an undergraduate degree or post-graduate diploma/Masters programme to prepare students to become dynamic occupational therapists to develop the future of the profession. See Table 1.1 below for the overall outcomes.

Table 1.1 Overall outcomes

The overall outcomes are:
The development of students into competent, reflective occupational therapists able to: • adapt and respond to current and future patterns of service delivery • analyse, select, adapt and use occupation and activity as therapeutic tools • adopt a problem solving approach to service users' needs • use theoretical frameworks of occupational therapy to guide and inform practice • understand and use the principles of evaluation and research to ensure best practice • view the delivery of occupational therapy in an holistic manner working in partnership with the service user • continue self development throughout their professional life.

Practice education comprises a significant proportion of the curriculum in pre-registration education programmes. This is the practical element when students undertake their learning in an area of service provision. Students must have a range of experiences in a variety of settings which may include health, social care and the third sector (College of Occupational Therapists, 2008). Each placement has specific essential learning outcomes that must be achieved in order to progress through the programme and on to the next placement. Responsibility for assessment within these settings lies with the practice educator. This person is qualified to supervise students while they are on practice placement and has usually undergone some form of training offered by the Higher Education Institution (College of Occupational Therapists, 2008) (see Chapter 4 for details on APPLE accreditation and preparation of educators). The practice educator must be a qualified occupational therapist, however, in some settings, particularly role emerging, they may not be on-site (Hocking and Ness, 2002).

Practice education provides the opportunity for students to experience occupational therapy in practice, to develop their therapeutic skills and to communicate with service users, carers and colleagues. McKenna et al., (2001) suggest that practice placements provide students with valuable opportunities to adopt the core values of the occupational therapy profession and Kasar and Muscari (2000) support that they enable the ongoing development of professional behaviours. Practice education involves a dynamic partnership between the practice educator and the student. The student is responsible for taking up the learning opportunities on offer whilst the supervisor should ensure that all such opportunities are made available. It offers an opportunity for rehearsal and reflection on practice and complements academic studies. It allows the students to achieve competence in the reality of practice, supported and assessed by the practice placement educator. Practice education is the most effective arena for students to learn about working with service users and their carers, and is the appropriate sociocultural environment where professional competence can be assessed. (See Chapter 2 for further detail on socio-cultural focused learning.) Practice education is also an arena where the development of the profession is taking place. Occupational therapy practice is emerging into new and innovative areas, and students are able to identify and analyse the potential emerging roles through the forum of practice education. This is discussed in more detail in Chapter 8.

There should always be regular formal supervision in practice education where there needs to be a fair and non-judgemental exchange of ideas, reflections and realistic objective setting. Informal supervision should take place on an ad hoc basis to include briefing and debriefing of tasks carried out with service users.

A summary of the aims of practice education is presented in Table 1.2.

Table 1.2 Aims of practice education

The aims of practice education are to:
<ul><li>provide an opportunity to learn new techniques, further knowledge, and experience working with a variety of people and develop professional working relationships;</li><li>enable students to transfer learning of core knowledge and skills in new and contrasting situations;</li><li>integrate academic and practice education and ensure the transfer of individually identified learning needs supported by academic staff via tutorials before, during and after placement;</li><li>develop reflective skills within the workplace.</li></ul>

How Practice Education is Incorporated into the Curriculum

Practice education must form an integral part of the occupational therapy programme (HPC, 2009) so that practice informs curriculum content and in turn the students inform practice in addition to learning from it. The synthesis and integration of academic and placement based modules are essential for the education of a competent, inquiring and creative practitioner (Hocking and Ness, 2002).

Within the curriculum undergraduate, pre-registration students will study at levels 4, 5 and 6 in England, Wales and Northern Ireland (The Quality Assurance Agency for Higher Education, 2008) and 8, 9 and 10 in Scotland (QAA Scotland, 2001). The placement learning outcomes must progressively increase in complexity in order to reflect these levels and indicate the students developing knowledge and skills. There is an expectation that the students will take responsibility for their own learning and transfer knowledge and skills from one placement to the next in a developmental manner akin to andragogy principles (Knowles, 1984) (see Chapter 2 for further detail on learning theory).

Practice education comprises of a tripartite relationship between the university, the student and the placement educator. For this to be successful, all parties must contribute equally to the process. Figure 1.1 below illustrates the inter-relationship between all three parties.

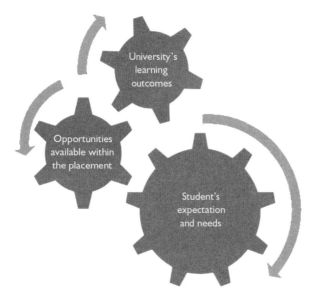

Figure 1.1 Inter-relationship between the three parties.

The university has set criteria (essential learning outcomes) that the educator must be familiar with and able to interpret into practical opportunities within the setting for the student to meet.

The student will also bring their individual expectations and needs to the learning process and these should be reflected back to the educator to be incorporated into the learning experience in order to meet the university's essential learning outcomes.

The three parties will also have specific learning and teaching styles/approaches that must be considered for an effective placement experience (see Chapters 3 and 4 for further information on learning styles and approaches). Figure 1.2 below illustrates the importance of fusing all three components in order to produce effective learning and teaching.

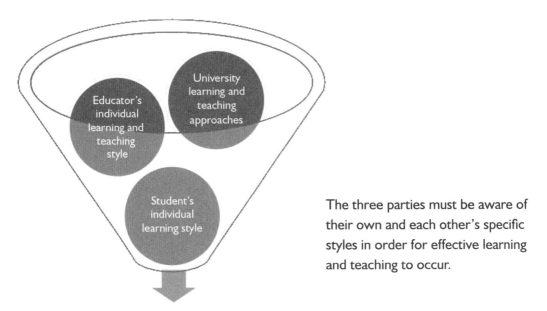

The three parties must be aware of their own and each other's specific styles in order for effective learning and teaching to occur.

Figure 1.2 Interaction of learning and teaching styles between key stakeholders

Funding Sectors, Areas of Practice and Service Settings

Occupational therapists can be employed in a wide diversity of settings, and the pool of potential employers across sectors is exponentially increasing. Figure 1.3 below seeks to illustrate the diversity of funding sectors that may employ occupational therapists, the areas of practice that they may work in and the multitude of service settings. The symbols linked to the areas of practice and service settings indicate the inter-relationship between the three areas. The figure illustrates that different service settings may be funded by different sectors, e.g. an occupational therapist working in a community team could be funded by Health, Local Authority or the third sector. Within each of these areas, the occupational therapist may work with people experiencing occupational interruption through a physical condition, mental health difficulty or a learning disability, and with individuals spanning the life cycle.

Funding sector

These are the bodies that provide the funding for the services. There are five key funding bodies that predominantly source services from occupational therapists.

Health and Social Care are the main areas employing occupational therapists. However the increasing number of role emerging placements in the third sector is indicative of the need to look outside the Health and Social Care placements (Cooper and Raine, 2009).

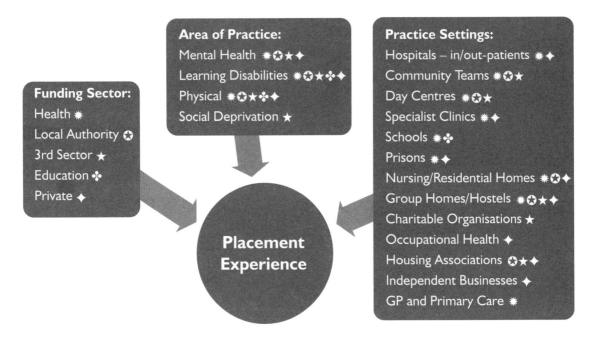

Figure 1.3 Funding sector, areas of practice and settings

Areas of practice

There are three key areas of practice: physical, mental health and learning disability, but there is an emerging role in the area of social deprivation. The majority of the five funding bodies finance services in the three main sectors.

Settings

This covers the diversity of areas in which occupational therapists may work. Within his/her career it is common for an occupational therapist to work in a range of settings and across sectors.

The Future

Figure 1.3 illustrates that the sectors providing occupational therapy services are wider than the traditional health and social care provision. These sectors, particularly the private and third sectors, continue to grow, especially in the changing face of provision of care in modern society. The profession of occupational therapy is creatively developing its scope of practice into new and innovative areas within all sectors, e.g. primary care GP practices. See Chapter 8 for more detail on the future development of occupational therapy practice and the role of practice education in this.

The changing demographics of British society will also need to be reflected in occupational therapy service provision, particularly in the growing elderly population. There is also a growing awareness and drive to promote healthy living; occupational therapists have a key role in promoting health through occupationally focused goals. Practice education needs to be proactive in anticipating these changes in society and ensuring students have opportunities to develop professional and entrepreneurial skills that prepare them for practice as an occupational therapist in modern society.

Summary

- Practice placements are a mandatory part of occupational therapy education with a requirement of a minimum of 1,000 assessed practice education hours.
- Placements provide the opportunity for students to transfer the theory learned in university into occupational therapy practice and vice versa.
- Effective placements rely upon a positive relationship between the university, the practice educator and the student.
- The diversity and opportunity for practice placements is wide ranging and the variety of settings available reflects the diversity and core skills required of occupational therapists.
- The profession continues to develop into innovative areas to reflect the needs of society.

Conclusion

This chapter has introduced practice education within the wider context of occupational therapy education. It has presented a range of sectors, areas of practice and settings where occupational therapy practice education occurs. The future direction for occupational therapy practice has also been briefly considered.

Reflective Questions

1. Consider how you have applied your academic learning to your placement experience and vice versa.
2. Reflect on the placements you have had and consider other areas that you would like to experience in order to develop your skills and knowledge.

References

Christiansen, A., and Bell, A. (2010) 'Peer learning partnerships: exploring the experience of pre-registration nursing students'. *Journal of Clinical Learning*, **19**: 803–810.

College of Occupational Therapists (2008). *College of Occupational Therapists Pre-Registration Education Standards* 3rd edition. London: College of Occupational Therapists.

Cooper, R. and Raine, R. (2009), 'Role emerging placements are an essential risk for the development of occupational therapy: The debate'. *British Journal of Occupational Therapy,* **72** (9): pp. 416–418.

Health Professions Council (2005) 'About Registration'. Available at http://www.hpc-uk.org/aboutregistration/ (accessed 26/04/12).

Health Professions Council (2009) *Standards of Education and Training Guidance*. London: Health Professions Council.

Hocking, C., and Ness, N.E. (2002) *Revised Minimum Standards for the Education of Occupational Therapists*. Perth: World Federation of Occupational Therapists.

Kasar, J., and Muscari, M.E. (2000) 'A conceptual model for the development of professional behaviours in occupational therapists'. *Canadian Journal of Occupational Therapy*. **67**(1): 42–50.

Knowles, K. (1984) *Andragogy in Action: Applying Modern Principles of Adult Education*. San Francisco: Jossey-Bass Inc.

McClure, P. (2004) 'Case Studies Occupational Therapy: An Overview of the Nature of the Preparation of Practice Education in Five Health Care Disciplines'. Available at www.practicebasedlearning.org (accessed 26/04/12).

McKenna, K., Scholtes, A.A., Fleming, J., and Gilbert, J. (2001) 'The journey through an undergraduate occupational therapy course: Does it change students' attitudes, perceptions and career plans?' *Australian Occupational Therapy Journal*. **48** (4): 157–169.

QAA Scotland (2001) *The Framework for Qualifications of Higher Education Institutions in Scotland*. Glasgow: QAA Scotland.

The Quality Assurance Agency for Higher Education (2008) *The Framework for Higher Education Qualifications in England, Wales and Northern Ireland*. Mansfield: The Quality Assurance Agency for Higher Education.

Turnock, C., Moran, P., Scammell, J., Mallik, M., and Mulholland, J. (2005) 'The preparation of practice educators: An overview of current practice in five healthcare disciplines'. *Work Based Learning in Primary Care*. **3**. 218–235.

Chapter 2
Theoretical Principles

Rachel Treseder and Tracey Polglase

Section 1

Introduction

In order to fully appreciate the significance of occupational therapy within the context of practice education today it is important to understand the development of the profession within the United Kingdom and the philosophical roots from which it stems. This chapter will aim to explore the history and philosophy of the profession and its development in practice education. This will culminate in current practice and cultural developments. The chapter will then conclude with an in-depth critical analysis of learning theories and approaches to guide practice.

History and Philosophy

The history and development of occupational therapy is a fascinating journey to trace due to its inextricable link to society and demographic changes within the last century. It would seem that the concept of occupation for health lends itself to a constantly evolving paradigm largely influenced by changes in society, and theoretical developments emerging from new research findings (Creek and Lawson-Porter, 2007).

In 1922 Dr. Adolf Meyer, a professor of psychiatry in the United States of America, expertly summarised the true value of occupation to health in his paper entitled 'A Philosophy of Occupation Therapy' (Meyer, 1922). This revolutionary and yet simplistic acknowledgement of the value of work and occupation in the adaptation to illness and disease, reflected decades of his work that was key in framing the use of occupation as therapy that has evolved to the profession that we know today.

The profession of occupational therapy emerged within the United Kingdom during the early decades of the twentieth century although arguably the use of occupation for health can be traced back to early historical writings prior to this (Wilcock, 2001; Marcil, 2007). In 1917 the profession was officially named 'occupational therapy' in America, closely followed two years later in Britain, and in 1925 the first trained occupational therapist was employed in the United Kingdom.

The social and political climate of this era greatly influenced the development of the profession. There had been an evolving recognition of the relationship between occupation and health and the Second World War served to increase the demand for therapeutic staff due to a greater need for rehabilitation. In the 1940s this unfamiliar concept of rehabilitation was increasingly viewed as fashionable in medical circles. This, along with the concept of holism, was soon aligned with the profession of occupational therapy, and the therapeutic value of occupation in the rehabilitative process. The establishment of the National Health Service in this decade was also significant in the future employment of occupational therapists.

The decades that followed witnessed a gradual evolution in the employment of occupational therapists in the public sector with the emphasis on rehabilitation. These were largely evident in physical hospitals and rehabilitation centres. The emerging paradigm of occupational therapy continued to evolve with the importance of principles such as client-centredness, enablement and working towards independence featuring strongly in the rehabilitative process. There was also significant value placed in the healing effects of community and groups of patients working together in therapeutic environments. There were new areas of practice that emerged during this era: palliative care and health promotion were just two where occupational therapy was beginning to be acknowledged as having a significant role.

As the profession of occupational therapy was becoming more recognised, an increasing number of therapists were being educated. As occupational therapy education evolved, so did the development of practice education – the practical element of training as an occupational therapist.

Developments in Practice Education

The importance of the practical element of occupational therapy education is illustrated in the establishment of Dorset House, the first School of Occupational Therapy in 1930 in Bristol. This school emerged from a nursing home for female patients with 'neurotic' or 'psychotic' disorders. Within this school the practical application of therapeutic activity was integral to the student's learning, as Dr Elizabeth Casson, a pioneer of occupational therapy in the United Kingdom, worked hard to develop a community integrating staff, patients and occupational therapy students. This 'holistic community' illustrates the importance of the practical element of the education of occupational therapists and the benefits of learning alongside patients (Wilcock, 2002).

The ratio of practical work to class based learning was significantly higher in the formative years of occupational therapy education. The six-month course offered by the Maudsley Hospital in London (which was the second institution of occupational therapy education in the UK) in the 1930s consisted of a six and a half-day week, three of which were spent with patients at the Maudsley.

More training schools opened and education developed in the decades to follow. From the 1950s students were required to complete 1440 hours of practical placements and by the 1970s a three-year course had been established. The placements were in a range of clinical areas where 'treatment of abnormality or adaptation to disability was the aim' (AOT undated in Wilcock, 2002, p. 244).

The education of occupational therapists was also being driven by the development of international standards. In 1952 the World Federation of Occupational Therapists was founded and one of the key documents at this time was the 'Establishment of a Programme for the Education of Occupational Therapists' which was published in 1958 (Hocking and Ness, 2002). The overarching aim at this point was to provide guidance for those countries that did not have an occupational therapy educational programme at that time.

Over the last five decades these standards have been revised and adapted to reflect changing practice and occupational therapy terminology and techniques. The current standards (Hocking and Ness 2002) were in response to countries requiring clearer guidance on the development and monitoring of educational programmes, and interestingly the perceived need for more flexibility in curriculum content and practice education (Hocking and Ness, 2002).

Some of the most noteworthy aspects of the standards in relation to practice education are the minimum requirements of 1000 hours of assessed practice education that must be completed within the programme and the depth and breadth of experiences that this needs to encompass. The most recent standards also acknowledge the new and emerging areas of practice for occupational therapy and the validity of the learning experience that this can provide for the student (Hocking and Ness, 2002). Developments are summarised in Table 2.1 below.

Table 2.1 Significant dates in the development of practice education

1930s	The first occupational therapy school was opened in Dorset House, Bristol by Dr Elizabeth Casson. This 'holistic community' optimised the therapeutic environment for educational purposes.
1936	Work-based practice was offered to staff within the Maudsley Hospital, London, to train as 'Occupation Nurses'. The practical element was almost 50% of this 6-month course.
1950s – 1970s	The Association of Occupational Therapists was founded. Regulations for training were set by the Association rather than individual educational institutions until the 1980s.
1952	Placements had to cover 1440 hours. Students had to reach a 'satisfactory' standard in hospital placements, with patients experiencing both physical and mental disorders.

1958	The World Federation of Occupational Therapists (WFOT) was founded.
1974	'Establishment of a Programme for the Education of Occupational Therapists' was published by WFOT.
1978	'Establishment of a Programme for the Education of Occupational Therapists' was published by WFOT.
1980s	The British Association of Occupational Therapists (BAOT) was formed.
1984	The BAOT formed the College of Occupational Therapists, who were primarily involved in the professional and educational aspects of occupational therapy.
2002	Placements had to cover 1200 hours within the UK, standards set by the College of Occupational Therapists.

Specifications for Fieldwork were included in an updated version of the 'Recommended Minimum Standards for the Education of Occupational Therapists' by WFOT. These included the minimum 1000 hours of practice education that needed to be completed by all students.

Current educational standards continue to maintain the minimum 1000 hours of practice education, with some flexibility in where these placements can now take place.

Current Practice/Cultural Developments

The brief history of the profession that has been mapped in this chapter has served to illustrate the reciprocal link between society and the development of the profession. This continues today; within the United Kingdom there are a number of drivers that influence the development of occupational therapy and the education of occupational therapists, whether professional, political, national or international (see Table 2.2).

Table 2.2 Current drivers impacting on the curriculum

Professional

- **Ongoing focus on occupation.**
- **Values and beliefs in occupation for health and well-being.**
- **Client-centred practice.**
- **Evidence-informed/based practice and sharing of such evidence.**
- **Developments of practice-driven research career pathways.**
- **Self-reliant practitioners.**
- **Reflective and reflexive practitioners.**

- Flexible and adaptable practitioners.
- Inter-professional, multi-professional and interagency working.
- Autonomy and accountability for professional work.
- Lifelong learning.
- Clarity about the uniqueness of occupational therapy.
- Development of the talents of occupational therapists in leadership, entrepreneurship, negotiation skills and business acumen.
- Generation and use of outcome measures to recognise the impact of occupational therapy.

Political

- The personalisation agenda. Increased expectations and purchasing power of service users.
- The significant changes in healthcare provision.
- Increasing research capacity and funding streams to promote the development of research capacity at Masters and Doctoral levels.
- Increased emphasis on health promotion.
- Emphasis on public health.
- Promotion of telecare and telehealth.
- Strengthened political awareness and activity to develop occupational therapy practice.
- Expansion of practice to address the needs of individuals, groups, communities and populations.
- Community-based rehabilitation.
- Government return-to-work agenda.
- Active ageing policies.
- Modernisation of allied health professions careers.
- Social inclusion: universal access to facilities.
- Widening participation in higher education.
- Marketing of the profession.
- Recovery model in mental health.
- Safeguarding.
- Better healthcare, well-being and quality of life for people with a learning disability.

National

- **Health Professions Council (HPC) *Standards of Education and Training* (2007).**
- **HPC *Standards of Proficiency* (2007).**
- **HPC *Code of Conduct* (2007).**
- **Increased community working.**
- **Increased flexibility in working patterns across a seven-day week.**
- **Increased work in the voluntary and independent sectors.**
- **Changing population demographics.**
- **Commissioning of competency based packages.**

International

- **Enhanced public health agenda.**
- **Standards of the World Federation of Occupational Therapists (Hocking and Ness 2002).**
- **International Classification of Function, Disability and Health (ICF).**
- **The TUNING of curricula across Europe.**
- **Internationalisation of curricula.**
- **Increased global mobility of occupational therapists.**

(College of Occupational Therapists, 2009, p. 14)

In 2009 the College of Occupational Therapists acknowledged these changes and asserted that in order to remain relevant and valued by society, changes needed to be made to the profession through three transformative processes:

1. The transformation of aspects of service users' lives through engagement in occupation.

2. The transformation of students into effective practitioners.

3. The transformation of the profession in response to changing contexts of service delivery.

(College of Occupational Therapists, 2009 p. 5)

These three components of transformation are seemingly separate and yet very much connected. The focus of this chapter, and indeed this book is on the second process – the transformation of students into effective practitioners. Yet it is with the overt acknowledgment that this particular transformational process cannot be achieved without the interplay of the service users and changing contexts of service delivery.

Current Context of Service Delivery

The last decade has witnessed a number of significant changes in the context of the arena in which occupational therapists are working. There are multiple reasons for this which can be attributed to demographic changes, government drivers and social factors (Creek 2003). There are currently almost 31,000 occupational therapists registered with the Health Professions Council (HPC, 2010) and there have been a number of developments in new and emerging areas that occupational therapists are now working in, as well as the traditional health and social care sectors.

One of the largest areas that occupational therapists are breaking new ground in is the voluntary third sector. Some of these settings include homeless hostels, youth charities, supported housing and learning disability workshops. It can be argued that practice education has had a significant role in the development and promotion of occupational therapy in these new and emerging areas (Cooper and Raine, 2009). This will be explored in more depth in relation to practice education in Chapter 8.

With the increasing changes in the contexts of employment of occupational therapists contributing to the complexity of intervention that is occupational therapy, it is evident that the transformation of students into effective practitioners is more crucial than ever. Practice education is a key component in the contribution to this, and the remainder of this chapter will focus on key learning theories that contribute to this transformational process.

Section 2

When considering learning theories there is much debate as to their categorisation. This section will present these theories in relation to the individual and the socio-cultural context. Analysis of the views on whether there is a distinction between the way adults learn (andragogy) and the way children learn (pedagogy) will be presented. A number of learning theories will be critiqued and applied to scenarios.

Bleakley (2006) distinguishes between learning theories that focus upon the individual (Knowles, 1980; Boud, 1987 and Kolb, 1984) and those that consider the sociocultural context of learning (Engestrom, 1987 and Sfard, 1998).

Individual Focused Learning Theories

Knowles (1980) is a key theorist in relation to adult learning theory. He draws strict distinctions between the way adults learn (andragogy) and the way children learn (pedagogy). Knowles has suggested that experiential learning is also a component of andragogy. Kolb (1984 p. 26b) has defined experiential learning as 'the process whereby knowledge is created through the transformation of experience'.

This book is written for, and focuses on, issues impacting on adult learning therefore it will focus on this aspect through the rest of the chapter.

Characteristics of adult learners (Knowles, 1984) have been summarised in Table 2.3.

Table 2.3 Characteristics of adults learners

Self Concept	As a person matures his/her self concept moves from one of being a dependent personality towards one of being a self directed human being.
Experience	As a person matures he/she accumulates a growing reservoir of experience that becomes an increasing resource for learning.
Readiness to Learn	As a person matures his/her readiness to learn becomes orientated increasingly to the development of tasks of his/her social roles.
Orientation to Learning	As a person matures his/her time perspective changes from one of postponed application of knowledge to immediacy of application, and accordingly his/her orientation towards learning shifts from one of subject centredness to one of problem centredness.

Knowles *et al.*, (2005) have developed Knowles' original work and added two further characteristics: 'The Need to Know' and 'Motivation'.

However there are other theorists who adopt a less purist style and suggest that both children and adults respond better to a more eclectic approach with methods associated with pedagogy and andragogy. Davenport's (1993) influential article argues that the distinction between the two is unfounded and lacks conceptual basis and empirical evidence. Adults entering education often have varying learning styles and strategies, however they can also require direction and guidance more akin to pedagogic principles. This is most evident when adults are insecure in their knowledge and lack confidence in their abilities. Adult learning is also not restricted to an academic activity within a university with the aim of achieving an award. Adults, like children are learning constantly through the experiences they are exposed to. Rogers (2003) terms this task conscious or acquisition learning. In a practice setting therapists often take on the role of educator or facilitator with service users. This may involve adopting an eclectic approach depending on the service user's requirements.

Skill Acquisition

Learning is ultimately about knowledge and skill acquisition. The theory and practise of skill acquisition has been documented in the literature. Dreyfus and Dreyfus (1980 cited in Benner 1982) produced the Dreyfus Model of Skill Acquisition; this describes five levels of proficiency the learner passes through during the learning process:

1. Novice
2. Advanced beginner
3. Competent
4. Proficient
5. Expert

Table 2.4 Application of model to practice

Dreyfus Model of Skill Acquisition	Application to Practice
1. Novice	Student
2. Advanced Beginner	Newly qualified staff
3. Competent	Newly qualified staff
4. Proficient	Experienced Band 6/Senior Practitioners
5. Expert	Clinical Specialists/Managers

In viewing this as a journey through the occupational therapy career, the student would be at the novice stage at the beginning of the occupational therapy programme, newly qualified therapists are at the advanced beginner/competent standard. Experienced band 6/senior practitioners are at the proficient and clinical specialists and managers at the expert level. However therapists can move up and down these levels according to their career pathway, e.g. expert level practitioners who move into education may move down a number of levels initially.

Abela (2009) presents an alternative to Dreyfus and Dreyfus (1980) with four stages for the learner:
1. Dependent
2. Interested
3. Involved
4. Self directed.

Abela suggests that the teaching style needs to match the learner's stage in order for learning to be successful. (See Chapter 4 for further information on learning styles.) If there is disparity this is likely to have a negative impact on the student's motivation to learn. Motivation has been highlighted by a number of writers as an important factor in the learning process.

Skill acquisition for occupational therapy students is predominantly achieved in practice. Bleakley's (2006) study in medical education presents Lave and Wenger's (1991) idea on 'cognitive apprenticeship' where it stresses that as novices learn the job and develop expertise they also 'think' and 'recount' the job. This is akin to transformative learning where clear elements of critical reflection are evident. This conscious focus on learning has been described by Rogers (2003) as learning conscious or formalised learning

Transformational Learning

Munro Turner (2004 p. 2) defines learning in three loops, see Figure 2.1. The three loops signify complexity of learning according to the level of thinking and change that comes from the action. He argues that the triple loop is the most complex because individual identity is formed and perceptions are changed at this level. This is defined as Transformational Learning.

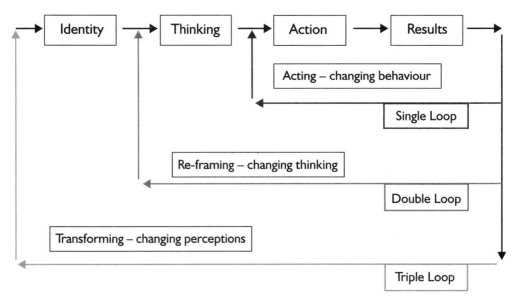

Figure 2.1 Three levels of learning

Mezirow initially introduced the concept of transformational learning in 1978 and defines it as:

> The process by which we transform problematic frames of reference (mindsets, habits of mind, meaning perspectives) – sets of assumption and expectation – to make them more inclusive, discriminating, open, reflective and emotionally able to change (Mezirow, 2006 p. 26)

Mezirow (2000) suggested a ten-step process of transformational learning. Table 2.5 illustrates the application of Mezirow (2000) and Munro Turner's (2004) models of transformational learning for a student undertaking a role emerging placement.

Transformational learning emphasises the use of reflection. As can been seen from the example (Table 2.5) reflection played a key role in the student's learning. Reflective practice is considered to be a key component of professional practice for therapists and in evidencing Continuing Professional Development (CPD). It is essential in both re-registration for the Health and Care Professions Council

(HCPC) and Accreditation of Practice Placement Educators (APPLE). The term reflection is often used by students and therapists but the process can be superficial e.g. thinking for 10 minutes about a particular piece of practice. This is possibly due to the organisational restrictions which emphasise practice and concrete output rather than reflection with ill defined output. This superficial process does not lead to a change in perception and practice unless there is a depth to the reflection. For this to occur critical reflection is required. Brookfield (1987, p. 87) defines critical reflection as 'reflecting on the assumptions underlying ours and others' ideas, and contemplating alternative ways of thinking and living'. Reflection will be further explored in Chapter 4 where specific models will be presented.

Table 2.5 Application of two models of transformational learning
(Mezirow, 2000 and Munro Turner, 2004)

10 Step Process of Transformational Learning (Mezirow 2000)	Three Levels of Learning Model (Munro Turner 2004)	Application of Model to a Student going on a Role-Emerging Placement.
1. Experience a disorientating dilemma	Single loop	First day the student is exposed to the setting and the personnel. All is new and unfamiliar with no set OT framework.
2. Undergo self examination	Single loop	The student reflects on his/her role and the expectations of him/her. The student may also question whether he/she can work in this setting and what he/she has to offer.
3. Conduct a deep assessment of personal role assumptions and alienation created by new role	Single/Double loop	The student may complete a reflective journal log highlighting their personal and professional values, beliefs and assumptions. This activity develops cognitive processing.
4. Share and analyse personal discontent and similar experiences with others	Single/Double loop	Issues discussed and analysed in supervision.
5. Explore options for new ways of acting	Double loop	As the student begins to develop confidence and skills he/she is able to select and justify suitable OT assessments and interventions. The student will be beginning to define his/her role and how he/she fits into the team.

6. Build competence and self confidence in new roles	Double loop	Practice in the skills through the placement increases competence and confidence. This will be further supported by positive feedback from colleagues, tutors and service users.
7. Plan a course of action	Double loop	The student becomes more autonomous in his/her practice and clinical reasoning is evident. The student's role is clearly defined in the organisation.
8. Acquire knowledge and skills for action	Double loop	Further practice, attendance at tutorials, joint working and research.
9. Try new roles and assessment feedback	Double/Triple loop	Following regular practical experience the student will receive informal and formal feedback from educator, service users and tutors. This will inform the student of his/her level of performance and assist him/her in developing practice skills. Areas of future development in placement highlighted in learning contract and discussed in supervision.
10. Reintegrate into society with a new perspective	Triple loop	At the end of the placement the student will go back to university with a new level of knowledge and skill that can be shared with people they interact with and the skills and knowledge will be transferable into future practice.

Socioculturally Focused Learning

Sfard (1998) distinguished between 'acquisition' and 'participatory' learning, where acquisition is about individual's knowledge reproduction through information seeking and participatory learning describes collaborative knowledge production within a community setting. In participatory learning the individual is involved in knowledge development but more importantly how to synthesise that within the context of the environment where they are learning. This model also covers the complexity of learning the values, beliefs and assumptions of the social organisation. Students need to adopt a sociocultural focused approach on placement. Not only do they need to know the practice issues, but also undergo professional socialisation into the values, beliefs and philosophy of the profession) and the systems, hierarchies and expectations, which Alsop and Ryan (1996) refer to as organisational socialisation.

Bleakley (2006) describes this style of learning within a socio-cultural approach. He argues that the learner is merely one aspect within a dynamic unstable activity system. In order for learning to happen there needs to be flexibility. As in change theory, if one element changes this has an impact on all other aspects (Hearle and Polglase, 2005). Engelstrom (1987) is a key theorist in the field of activity theory. He studied work based learning within specific systems across intersectoral organisations. This model of learning is particularly relevant for interprofessional settings as it involves analysing elements that are shared, e.g. the service user, and boundary crossing, e.g. understanding of others' roles and elements of generic responsibility.

Lawrie (2007, p. 55) developed a new model of learning for mature students, 'The Learning Tree'. This considers intrinsic and extrinsic factors that impact upon the learning process, but emphasises the holistic and humanistic focus. This model clearly fits within the socio-cultural focused framework (see Figure 2.2, p. 24).

To summarise this chapter a new model of professional development for occupational therapists is presented (see Figure 2.3, p. 25). This aims to incorporate the elements of development in a sequential pyramid while also accepting that external influences will impact upon the process to either facilitate or inhibit the development. That is, a supportive culture within an organisation that encourages supervision and peer mentorship can facilitate professional development, whereas an environment that focuses only on output figures and is not directed to support the staff is likely to inhibit staff development.

The first level focuses on the key elements of skill acquisition, both profession specific and generic. To support this there is also a requirement to develop theoretical knowledge in relation to professional theory, learning and reflection. CPD activities will assist the professional in making sense of these. This level will be developed predominantly through the student and newly qualified stages.

The second level focuses on evaluation. The student/therapist begins to link the theory to practice in relation to both professional and reflective issues. This will begin in the later stages of the student's training but develop in the early stages of the professional's practice.

The third level focuses on synthesis. This relies on a sound level of clinical reasoning built upon well developed knowledge and skills. It also requires the therapist to have skills of reflexivity and highly developed skills of self awareness in relation to their knowledge, skills and practice. These combined skills will be used to create evidence-based practice (EBP) through the research process. This should be clearly evidenced by senior therapists.

Once all the elements are soundly in place it will lead to the top tier where the focus is on clinical analysis. The therapist is expected to be a critical thinker and expert practitioner.

Each level needs to be achieved in order to move successfully to the next level. Insufficient depth and understanding of all components in the preceding level when moving to the next will lead to unstable foundations and weaknesses in assimilating the information at more complex levels.

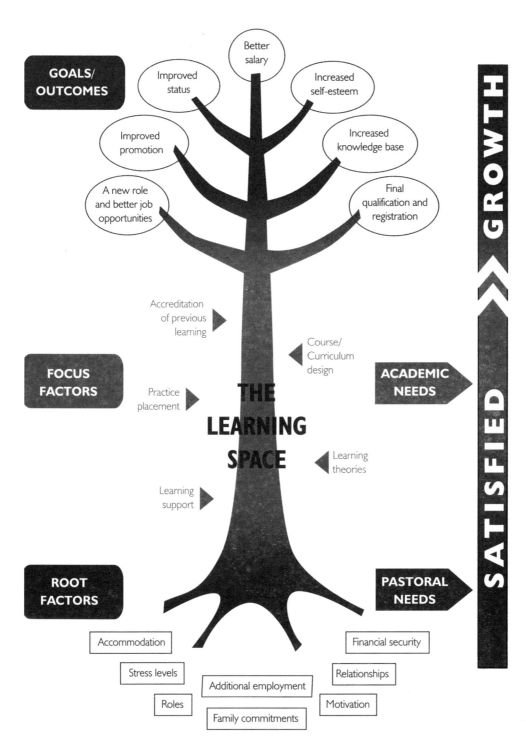

Figure 2.2 The Learning Tree – A model of learning for mature students

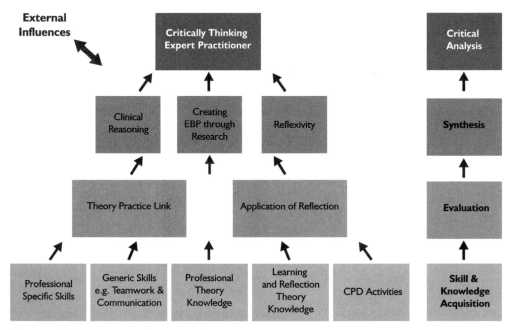

Figure 2.3 Pyramid of professional development

Conclusion

This chapter has presented an overview of the history and development of occupational therapy in the United Kingdom, from the early decades of the twentieth century to the present, drawing attention to the emphasis on practical work in occupational therapy education. It then focused on the development of practice education and the various drivers impacting on the curriculum, culminating in the current context of service delivery.

The second half of the chapter presented material to support students and occupational therapists to recognise key learning theories and apply them to personal and professional development. This included discussion of the distinctive features of adult learners, the stages of learning and proficiency, and the concepts of transformational learning and socioculturally focused learning. Lastly we presented a model of the levels of professional development for occupational therapists, relating the theoretical insights previously discussed to the specific context of occupational therapy.

Reflective Questions

1. Occupational therapy has come a long way since its inception, where do you see the key developments in the next decade?

2. How do you see yourself in being involved in the development of the profession?

3. How do you feel applying one of the models presented in this chapter would assist you in critiquing your personal development to a greater degree?

References

Abela, J. (2009) 'Adult learning theories and medical education: A review'. *Malta Medical Journal,* **21** (1): 11–18.

Alsop, A., and Ryan, S. (1996) *Making the Most of Fieldwork Education: A Practical Approach.* Cheltenham: Nelson Thorne.

Benner, P. (1982) 'From novice to expert'. *American Journal of Nursing,* **82**: 402–7.

Bleakley, A. (2006) 'Broadening conceptions of learning in medical education: The message from teamworking'. *Medical Education,* **40**: 150–7.

Boud, D. (1987) *Developing Student Autonomy in Learning.* London: Routledge Falmer.

Brookfield, S. (1987) *The Modern Practice of Adult Education: Post Modern Critique.* Albany: State University of New York Press.

College of Occupational Therapists (2009) 'Curriculum Guidance for Pre-Registration Education'. London: College of Occupational Therapists.

Cooper, R., and Raine, R. (2009) 'Role emerging placements are an essential risk for the development of occupational therapy: The debate'. *British Journal of Occupational Therapy,* **72** (9): 416–18.

Creek, J. (2003) 'Occupational Therapy Defined as a Complex Intervention'. London: College of Occupational Therapists.

Creek, J., and Lawson-Porter, A. (2007) *Contemporary Issues in Occupational Therapy: Reasoning and Reflection.* Chichester: John Wiley & Sons.

Davenport, J. (1993) 'Is there a way out of the andragogy morass?' In M. Thorpe, R. Edwards. and A. Ranson. *Culture and Process of Adult Learning.* London: Routledge. pp.109–17.

Engestrom, Y. (1987) *Learning by Expanding: An Activity–Theoretical Approach to Development Research.* Helsinki: Orienta-Konsultit Oy.

Health Professions Council (2010) *Statistics – Current.* Available at www.hpc-uk.org (accessed 26/04/12).

Hearle, D., and Polglase, T. (2005) 'Working within a process of change' in T.J. Clouston and L. Westcott, *Working in Health and Social Care: An Introduction for Allied Health Professionals.* London: Elsevier Churchill Livingstone pp. 41–57.

Hocking, C. and Ness, N.E. (2002) *Revised Minimum Standards for the Education of Occupational Therapists.* Perth: World Federation of Occupational Therapists.

Knowles, M.S. (1980) *The Modern Practice of Adult Education: From Pedagogy to Andragogy.* San Francisco: Jossey-Bass Inc.

Knowles, M.S. (1984) *Andragogy in Action: Applying Modern Principles of Adult Education.* San Francisco: Jossey-Bass Inc.

Knowles, M.S., Holton, E.F. and Swanson, R.A. (2005) *The Adult Learner.* London: Elsevier Butterworth Heinemann.

Kolb, D. (1984) *Experiential Learning: Experience as the Source of Learning and Development.* Englewood Cliffs: Prentice Hall.

Lave, J., and Wenger, E. (1991) *Situated Learning: Legitimate Peripheral Participation.* Cambridge: Cambridge University Press.

Lawrie, C. (2007) *The Factors Impacting upon the Learning Needs of Mature Students Involved in Undergraduate and Post Graduate, Pre-registration Courses in the United Kingdom for Professions Allied to Medicine. A Literature Review.* MSc. Cardiff University. (Unpublished dissertation).

Marcil, W.M. (2007) *Occupational Therapy: What it is and How it Works.* New York: Thomson Delmar Learning.

Meyer, A. (1922) 'A philosophy of occupational therapy'. *Archives of Occupational Therapy* (1): 1–10.

Mezirow, J. (1997) 'Transformational learning: Theory to practice'. *New Directions in Adult and Continuing Education* 74: 5–12.

Mezirow, J. (2000) *Learning as Transformation: Critical Perspectives on Theory in Progress.* San Francisco: Jossey-Bass Inc.

Mezirow, J. (2006) 'An overview of transformative learning'. In P. Sutherland and J. Crowther, (Eds) *Lifelong Learning: Concepts and Contexts*. Abingdon: Routledge. pp. 24–38.

Munro Turner, M. (2004) *Transformational Learning*. Available at http://www.mentoringforchange.co.uk (accessed 26/04/12).

Rogers, A. (2003) *What is the Difference? A New Critique of Adult Learning and Teaching*. Leicester: NIACE.

Sfard, A. (1998) 'On two metaphors for learning and on the danger of choosing just one'. *Educational Research*, **27**: 4–13.

Wilcock, A. (2001) *Occupation for Health: Volume 1. A Journey from Self Health to Prescription*. London: College of Occupational Therapists.

Wilcock, A. (2002) *Occupation for Health: Volume 2. A Journey from Prescription to Self Health*. London: College of Occupational Therapists.

Chapter 3

Preparation of Students for Placement

Maria Clarke and Rachel Treseder

Introduction

Practice placements can be both exciting and anxiety provoking experiences for students (Tan *et al.*, 2004). Preparation for placements can help make students feel more in control and equipped for the learning experiences available to them. Although it would be impossible to identify everything that needs to be addressed in relation to placement, this chapter will provide some guidance on how a student should prepare for this essential element of the programme. It will inform the students of the requirements prior to placement, e.g. Criminal Records Bureau check, satisfactory occupational health screening together with training requirements, e.g. Moving and Handling and Basic Life Support. Practical issues will be identified, e.g. the need for business insurance when using a car on placement, finding accommodation, travel expenses, dress code requirements, etc.

Checks

Criminal Records Bureau check

Prior to starting the course, the student will have been asked to complete an Enhanced Criminal Records Bureau (CRB) application. This is a mandatory requirement for all people who are likely to be working with children, young people or vulnerable adults (CRB, 2011a). Clearance from the CRB is essential before any student can undertake a practice placement so prompt completion of the application is strongly advised. When filling in the application form, information provided must be accurate, legible and complete to avoid delay in processing.

Once clearance has been achieved, it usually lasts for the duration of the student's programme. The student will be asked to sign a declaration at the start of each academic year confirming there are no changes to his/her clearance status. Any changes to the status could ultimately impact on the student's ability to gain registration with the Health and Care Professions Council (HCPC) and might result in him/her being unable to practice as an occupational therapist following graduation.

Health screening

All students accepted for occupational therapy courses throughout the United Kingdom will undergo a review of their health through completing a health-screening questionnaire and attending an occupational health appointment. This will ensure students are fit for practice and will provide opportunities for them to ensure all immunisations are up to date. Some placement settings may ask the student to provide evidence of health status and may even ask for an assessment with the local occupational health services.

Students are also able to access continued support for any health issues through accessing student support services. The university website will provide contact details of the student support services available locally.

Additional Training in Preparation for Placement

There are a number of additional issues that are usually addressed prior to practice placement commencing. Universities may offer practical training in manual handling, basic life support and managing challenging behaviour. Many practice settings also require that students have an understanding of minimal handling (also referred to as manual handling) and basic life support (first aid). The Health and Safety Executive (HSE, 2011a) provide access to a range of materials that might be a useful resource for students. A leaflet can be downloaded that offers advice on basic first aid from http://www.hse.gov.uk/pubns/indg347.pdf (HSE, 2011b). There is also advice available on manual handling regulations and how these influence practice for students on placement. A useful guide to manual handling best practice can be accessed from http://www.hse.gov.uk/pubns/indg143.pdf (HSE, 2006).

Students need to familiarise themselves with local policies and procedures relating to health and safety within the workplace as these may vary from one placement setting to another. This information will usually be included as part of the placement induction with the practice educator.

Other Practical Issues

There are a number of other practical issues that may need to be considered prior to starting the practice placement. See Table 3.1 below.

Table 3.1 Other things to consider

Issue	Consideration/Solution
Sufficient insurance cover for using personal car during practice placement	Universities access a wide range of practice settings for student placements, many of which are community based. Depending on the timing of the placement (e.g. towards the end of the studies) some educators will encourage students to use their car to visit service users or other settings. It is therefore strongly advisable to ensure there is business insurance cover for doing this. The student should check with the insurance provider that he/she is covered for business use when using his/her car.
Accommodation provision if the placement is away from either home or term address	Students should be provided with details of the location of the placement well in advance of it starting. Some placements are likely to be away from either home or term address and will require that the student resides in alternative accommodation for the duration of the placement. This may be arranged independently, via the university or via the educator.
Reimbursement of expenditure to cover cost of accommodation and additional travel	If the student is receiving a bursary, lives in rented accommodation and needs to stay in alternative accommodation for their placement he/she is entitled to claim back one of the accommodation costs (the cheaper of the two) from his/her sponsor. Some students will also be eligible to claim back any expenses incurred directly related to travel involved as part of the placement. The student will be required to provide proof of expenditure, e.g. bus tickets, receipts, etc. Each university will have an expenses claim form that needs to be completed.
Dress code for placement	It is important to adopt the dress code stipulated by the setting. This can be confirmed at the pre-placement meeting. Placements within an in-patient setting often require students to wear their uniform. If this is the case, ensure it is clean and ironed and follow any local policies relating to wearing it outside the workplace, i.e. for commuting. Community settings may not require uniform to be worn, but recommend smart casual dress. Keep jewellery to a minimum (other than stud earrings and a wedding band) and have comfortable footwear.

Placement Preparation

There will be an opportunity to explore many of these issues during pre-placement teaching sessions facilitated by members of the university teaching staff. Some of the subjects covered may include using learning contracts to guide learning, accessing learning resources, reflective practice, communication skills (both verbal and non-verbal) supervision and how policy and legislation influences practice as occupational therapists (see Chapter 4 for more information).

Communication with the Educator Prior to the Start of the Placement

When the placement details are confirmed the student should make contact with the placement educator. There are expectations of good practice in communicating with the educator. Initial contact should be made via telephone or email. At this point a request for a pre-placement visit at a mutually convenient time can be made.

Pre-placement visit

A pre-placement visit is advisable, but may not be possible if long distances are involved. When making an appointment for a pre-placement visit ensure the educator is given plenty of notice to schedule the visit into the diary. One to two weeks is advisable. This visit allows students to familiarise themselves with the route, transport, parking, etc. It also gives an opportunity to discuss with the educator specific aspects about the placement and to clarify any issues.

A curriculum vitae (CV) will give the educator further information. This can be sent to the educator prior to the pre-placement visit or given during the meeting.

If a visit is not possible a telephone call is advisable to discuss issues regarding the placement. A letter and CV should always be sent to the educator if a pre-placement visit is not possible.

Suggestions for content of the letter and CV are listed below.

Letter

When writing to the educator include a covering letter detailing the following:

- Full contact address (for them to write back)
- Confirmation of the placement dates and theme
- Request for relevant information, e.g.
  time of arrival,
  directions,
  accommodation details,
  whether or not uniform is worn,
  what preparatory work is needed,

what specific skills may be needed,

who the client group is,

which assessments, approaches or techniques are used most frequently.

Curriculum vitae

Together with the letter a current curriculum vitae (CV) is required. A CV may be written in a variety of ways but should include:

- name
- contact address, email and telephone number
- personal statement: Include information about yourself and the things you enjoy doing, e.g. interests and hobbies
- educational background/qualifications
- previous work experiences and relevant skills. You can also include voluntary work and caring activities
- relevant courses: e.g. work based, etc.
- college work completed: give an overview of what you have studied to date
- previous placements: Where these were, the types of setting, the service user groups, skills learnt, etc.

The CV is a way of giving the educator some relevant information to assist in planning the placement to suit the individual student's learning needs. It will need to be updated before every placement and will become the basis of the professional CV when applying for jobs. It will also be the basis of the professional portfolio, which is required in order to register as a practising occupational therapist (Health Act 1999). It is therefore worth the effort of getting it right.

Learning Contracts

Many universities use learning contracts to enable students to identify their learning needs within the context of the placement setting. They provide valuable opportunities to shape individual learning, whilst ensuring the essential learning outcomes of the placement are addressed. Learning contracts can offer a versatile tool from which an agreement can be negotiated between the student and the placement educator (Whitcombe, 2001). Learning contracts are effective in highlighting learning needs, the resources that can be accessed to facilitate this learning and criteria to evidence and validate the learning outcomes. In this way, the student will be able to tailor the learning experience so that it is individualised to his/her learning needs, thus optimising the overall practice placement experience (Kirke et al., 2007).

Accessing Learning Resources

There is a wide range of resources that can be accessed to inform learning. Text books, journals and the internet are all valuable resources. Another valuable learning resource is the practice placement educator and other professionals/support staff within the setting. Service users and their family/carers also will provide invaluable learning opportunities and feedback during the practice placement.

Creative use of resources and time will assist the student in meeting his/her learning needs, e.g. during quiet periods take some time to explore local resources that are available. Many placement settings have a student resource file available which might provide useful information. This can also be developed for future students. Some placement settings will have a library/learning resource centre offering full or partial access to the student.

Reflective Practice

Reflective practice is widely acknowledged within healthcare professional practice as a means of examining and analysing everyday working experiences in order to improve levels of competence, professional development and clinical reasoning (Clouder, 2000; Ronald *et a.l*, 2002). The skill of reflective practice should start as a student practitioner and develop over the time of the pre-registration course and into professional practice.

As with any new skill, the ability to reflect effectively needs to be practised in order to develop competence in the process. Reflecting on incidences experienced on placement gives the student the ideal opportunity to start developing this skill. There are a number of tools the student can use to assist in this process and several models of reflection have been developed that might be useful (see Chapter 4). Gibbs (1988) developed a popular model of reflection called the Cycle of Reflection. This model has a six-stage process for exploring and analysing events in order to identify an action plan to inform future practice.

Communication Skills (also see Chapter 5)

The ability to communicate both verbally and non-verbally is an essential skill for any healthcare professional. As occupational therapists, there is a duty to work in partnership with service users and their carer/s (COT, 2010a), which require effective verbal communication skills throughout the occupational therapy process. There is also a duty to maintain a written record '*of all that has been done for/with or in relation to a service user, including the clinical reasoning behind the care planning and provision*' (COT, 2010a, p. 19).

Assertive verbal communication skills are important when working within a multidisciplinary team. The university may use case study scenarios and role plays to enable the student to practise this prior to going out on placement, but ultimately, the student needs to present him/herself in a confident and professional manner.

Most practice settings have a preferred format for documenting service user records and writing reports. The student needs to familiarise him/herself with these methods and ensure his/her work is legible and objective. The College of Occupational Therapists (COT, 2010b) have developed standards for practice on record keeping and it would be useful to become acquainted with this document prior to starting placement. All written documentation produced by the student on placement needs to be countersigned by a qualified occupational therapist.

One key message in relation to any form of communication that relates to a service user is the need to 'safeguard confidential information' (COT, 2010a, p. 11). Failure to respect this could result in disciplinary action being taken.

Conclusion

This chapter has presented the practical elements that need to be considered and addressed prior to the student going on placement. It is essential that preparation is undertaken by the student, the university staff, and the educator in order for an effective placement to occur.

Reflective Questions

1. After reading this chapter what do you consider are the priorities for you to plan effectively for your next placement?
2. How could you develop assertive verbal communication skills in order to prepare yourself for placement?

References

Clouder, L. (2000) 'Reflective practice in physiotherapy education: A critical conversation.' *Studies in Higher Education*, **25**(2): 211–223.

College of Occupational Therapists (2010a) *Code of Ethics and Professional Conduct*. London: College of Occupational Therapists.

College of Occupational Therapists (2010b) *Professional Standards for Occupational Therapy and Guidance on Record Keeping*. London. College of Occupational Therapists.

Criminal Records Bureau (2011a) 'About CRB'. Available at http://www.crb.homeoffice.gov.uk/about_crb.aspx (accessed 26/04/12).

Gibbs, G. (1988) *Learning by Doing: A Guide to Teaching and Learning Methods*. Further Education Unit, Oxford Polytechnic, Oxford.

Health Act (1999) Available at www.legislation.gov.uk/ukpga/1999/8/contents (accessed 26/04/12).

Health and Safety Executive (2006) 'Getting to Grips with Manual Handling: A Short Guide.' Available at http://www.hse.gov.uk/pubns/indg143.pdf (accessed 26/04/12).

Health and Safety Executive (2011a) 'Health and Safety Executive (Home Page)'. Available at http://www.hse.gov.uk/index.htm (accessed 26/04/12).

Health and Safety Executive (2011b) 'Basic Advice on First Aid at Work'. Available at http://www.hse.gov.uk/pubns/indg347.pdf (accessed 26/04/12).

Kirke, P., Layton, N., and Sims, J. (2007) 'Informing fieldwork design: Key elements to quality in fieldwork education for undergraduate occupational therapy students.' *Australian Occupational Therapy Journal*, **54**(1): 13–22.

Ronald, M., Epstein, M.D., Edward, M., and Hundert, M.D. (2002) 'Defining and assessing professional competence' *Journal of the American Medical Association*, **287** (2): 226–235. Available at http://jama.ama-assn.org/cgi/content/full/287/2/226 (accessed 26/04/12).

Tan, K-P., Meredith, P., and McKenna, K. (2004) 'Predictors of occupational therapy students' clinical performance: An exploratory study. *Australian Occupational Therapy Journal*, **51**(1): 25–33.

Whitcombe, S.W. (2001) 'Using learning contracts in fieldwork education: The views of occupational therapy students and those responsible for their supervision.' *British Journal of Occupational Therapy*, **64**(11): 552–558.

Part 2

Knowledge and Skill Development on Placement

Chapter 4
The Learning Experience on Placement

Liz Cade and Tracey Polglase

Introduction

This chapter will present the roles and responsibilities of both the educator and the student whilst on placement. Within this chapter strategies to identify and develop learning styles for students whilst on placement will be presented, e.g. suggested tools for reflection. Further topics to be integrated within this chapter will include methods of assessment of the student, different models of supervision and support and processes for evaluating the experience

Roles and Responsibilities
The educator

Occupational therapists have a professional responsibility to facilitate and promote a learning culture in practice environments to provide experiential opportunities for students (COT, 2007, 2008, 2010; Health Professions Council, (HPC), 2008). Field (2004) suggests that for learning to make sense to students, it must be situated in real life contexts where they can legitimately participate. Educators require an understanding of their role and responsibilities and an ability to provide learning experiences to ensure quality placements that fulfil the needs of all students (COT, 2008; HPC, 2007, 2008; QAA, 2008). Each educator must have an in-depth understanding of the specific requirements and processes for placement education for students from individual universities to wholly fulfil their responsibilities (COT, 2010).

The practice educator is considered to be an experienced therapist predominantly working within health or social care who brings a high level of tacit knowledge and skill to the role (Cross et al., 2006). The decision to become a practice educator is usually considered to be appropriate a year or two post qualification. At this stage, knowledge has been consolidated and the therapist can then broaden and develop skills to encompass facilitation of the undergraduate learning with students, in addition to their professional role and clinical duties. Embracing this role clearly demonstrates the individual therapist's involvement in professional development and offers an invaluable contribution to the profession (Ledgerd, 2005; COT, 2010). The APPLE accreditation scheme (COT, 2006) was introduced as a nationally recognised route to becoming an accredited practice educator.

The practice educator role is complex and deemed to be one that encompasses that of being:

- a facilitator of learning
- a manager
- a mentor
- an assessor
- an evaluator and reflector.

(Best *et al.*, 2005; Cross *et al.*, 2006).

Each aspect of the role will now be considered and will draw upon the practicalities of achieving the role in practice. See Table 4.1 below.

Table 4.1 The roles and responsibilities of the educator

Role	Responsibilities: The educator needs to:
Facilitator of learning	Work in partnership with the student to identify the student's learning needs and methods of learning throughout the placement.
	Provide learning opportunities appropriate to the placement setting enabling the student to fulfil the expected learning outcomes (Morris, 2007).
	Provide a supportive environment where the student feels valued, where he/she has a sense of belonging with his/her own space to work and access resources.
	Ensure the student feels supported, understood and is able to fully engage in the learning process and search for their own identity (Myall *et al.*, 2008, Webb *et al.*, 2009).
Manager	Prior to the arrival of the student:
	Identify resources appropriate to the learning experience and provide an updated resource folder.
	Plan sessions and visits.
	Inform the student of expectations and practicalities (in terms of uniform/dress code, parking, prior reading, etc.).

	Be aware of policies and procedures and facilitate access to IT systems where appropriate.
	Plan specific training/induction which may be a mandatory requirement of the setting.
	During the placement:
	Ensure the student is given a full induction within the setting.
	Manage the practical, day to day requirements of the placement and student learning throughout the placement (Cross *et al.*, 2006; Brown and Kennedy Jones, 2005).
	Plan essential elements such as formal supervision on a weekly basis, half way visits, specific teaching sessions, etc.
	Ensure the final report and assessment documentation is completed according to the university's requirements.
	Continue to prioritise their caseload and provide appropriate practical learning opportunities.
	Collaborate with other professionals to optimise the student learning.
Mentor	Use knowledge, skills and attitudes to influence the development of students' professional identities.
	Provide pastoral, personal support to the student which can be vital to a successful outcome of a placement.
	Support the student to navigate their way through difficult decisions or situations by guiding their thinking and practice (Neugebauer and Evans-Brain, 2009; Duke 2004).
Assessor	Assess the knowledge and competencies of a student and whether they have successfully achieved the learning outcomes of the placement (McBurney, 2005; Gopee, 2010).
	Be a gatekeeper for the profession (Cross *et al.*, 2006).
	Convert university's outcomes into practical tasks where students can demonstrate the required standards of practice (Craik, 2009).
	Record evidence and document supervision throughout, so this can be drawn upon to explicitly explain why such an assessment outcome has been reached.

cont.

Evaluator and/or Reflector	Use the following tools in evaluation of the student:
	Evaluation forms (internal and those provided by the university).
	Feedback, discussion and supervision.
	Reflective tools and reflective models.
	Peer learning through educator support mechanisms.
	Mentorship.
	Critically analyse the positive and negative learning experiences and deepen his/her understanding of the learning experience and the outcome.
	Develop their skills, knowledge and ability to facilitate learning for future student placements (COT, 2008; HPC, 2008).

The student

The student also has a number of roles and responsibilities before, during and after they finish placement. It is essential that the student is aware of key policies that will impact upon their performance, e.g. *Code of Ethics and Professional Conduct* (COT, 2010) and *Guidance on Conduct and Ethics of Students* (HPC, 2009). Table 4.2 highlights specifically the responsibilities related to the two key roles of 'self-directed learner' and 'student practitioner'.

Table 4.2 The roles and responsibilities of the student

Role	Responsibilities: The student needs to:
Self-directed Learner	Be an active participant in the placement and work in partnership with the educator.
	Progress from initially being predominantly educator directed to independent and self-directed practice as he/she progresses through the academic levels of the degree.
	Investigate and explore learning opportunities available whilst on placement.
	Start enquiring about preparatory reading and key learning for inclusion in the learning contract at the pre-placement visit.
	Carry over learning needs from one placement to the next.
	Indicate if he/she has any learning difficulties which may impede progress whilst on placement. Discuss strategies and practical ways of overcoming the difficulties.

Student Practitioner	Demonstrate professional competence and reasoning in his/her practice as required to reach qualification (HPC, 2007). Holmes *et al.* (2010), suggest students begin this process through the acquisition of knowledge and skills, leading to its application in practice and finally consolidation with effective clinical reasoning.
	Link theory to practice.
	Develop professional identity and behaviour drawing upon the educator as a role model and from the cultural ethos within the placement setting (Duke, 2004, McIntosh, 2011).
	Observe the educator and others and discuss the clinical reasoning process using each learning opportunity to increase his/her expertise.
	Adhere to the professional standards and ensure ethical conduct throughout the placement (COT, 2010; QAA, 2007).
	Experience a range of placements, this will build through multiple learning experiences with the aim of achieving professional competence by the end of undergraduate study.
	Be mindful of his/her professional responsibility and have insight into his/her own level of competence. When faced with uncertainty and difficult clinical reasoning the student must always seek guidance and utilise supervision in an effective and constructive way to guide practice (COT, 2007, 2010).

The Collaborative Learning Process for the Student and Educator

Although the educator and the student have separate roles and responsibilities they must work together throughout the placement to ensure learning is optimised if the required learning outcomes are to be achieved. Therefore, the educator needs to be aware how the individual student learns as this is pivotal to the learning process (Cross *et al.*, 2006; Hulme and Hulme, 2011). The student and educator should be aware of their own learning styles and how these complement and conflict with one another. The importance of understanding adult learning theories such as andragogy (Fry *et al.*, 2003; Gopee 2010) and motivation to learn cannot be underestimated and has been discussed in depth in Chapter 2.

Understanding how learning occurs

Each individual brings their own approach to learning. At the start of the placement students and educators will find it beneficial to discuss preferred learning styles as this will enable the educator to facilitate the learning experience in a way that the student can understand and assist them in making the link between theory and practice (Fry et al., 2003). A specific tool such as a learning styles questionnaire can be completed to help direct the learning and in the formulation of the learning contract. For example:

- Honey and Mumford Learning Styles Questionnaire (Honey and Mumford, 2000) identifies four styles of learning: activist, pragmatist, reflector and theorist.

- Fleming (2010) also developed a learning styles questionnaire that identifies four types of learners: visual, auditory/aural, read/write and kinaesthetic. The questionnaire can be accessed and completed online via the following website:
  http://www.vark-learn.com/english/page.asp?p=questionnaire

It is important for the educator to recognise his/her own learning style. This can be achieved by completion of such a questionnaire. Where there are clear differences in how the student and educator learn progress can be impeded unless issues are taken into consideration, for example: demonstrating a practical skill using oral or visual instruction to facilitate learning, when the student may prefer to learn using a 'hands on' or kinaesthetic style. The skill of the educator is to adapt how they teach or facilitate tasks or experiences to meet the individual needs of the student.

Developing the learning contract

For many practice placements the use of a learning contract is an integral tool for ensuring the learning is focused, explicit and links theory to practice (Whitcombe, 2001; Matheson, 2003). The learning contract may form a key element to inform the assessment of the student competence and must therefore link to the specific placement outcomes. See Figure 4.1 below.

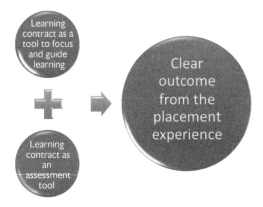

Figure 4.1 Multifaceted use of a learning contract

A learning contract also allows a student to:

- take responsibility for their own learning and show how they can demonstrate they have met the required competency level for each learning outcome or objective (Tsang et al., 2002).
- formulate their learning needs, usually within the first two weeks, in collaboration with the educator, who can guide and advise what resources, opportunities and experiences are available in the setting.
- guide practice and learning throughout the duration of the placement (Yeung et al., 2001).

A number of students are initially daunted by constructing their learning contract; some disregard its importance and contribute minimum effort to its formulation. Those who fully embrace the purpose of a well constructed contract find significant benefits as it serves to structure their learning and allows them to focus on how to achieve the placement outcomes. However, all students benefit from guidance to ensure the learning contract is realistic, achievable and explicit. If used in conjunction with supervision, the learning contract should guide the student to a successful completion of their placement.

Reflective learning and teaching

'Reflective practice is a critical component in the learning experience … allowing practitioners to develop in the real world setting'; making sense of what worked well and where it did not is crucial in development of clinical reasoning skills as a healthcare professional (Healey and Spencer, 2008, p. 23).

Reflection is an integral part of being an educator (Biggs, 2003). Being able to evaluate your own practice as a professional role model to students and being open to development and your own learning ensures a valued placement experience for students. Educators need to reflect on the positive and negative aspects of the placement, their facilitation and planning of the placement, and in their role of being supervisor, assessor and mentor. They need to question what more could be done to enhance student learning and seek an insight into their own professional performance (Craik, 2009). Students need to learn how to reflect, as they may not be a reflector by nature and so need to understand its importance in day-to-day practice. Therefore educators have to act as a role model to students allowing them to develop reflective skills and facilitate opportunities for the student to reflect upon their practice (Baird and Winter, 2005).

The use of reflective tools in conjunction with supervision enables the student to develop their reflective skills and may be of a formal, structured nature or informal.

Tools for reflection

- Reflective journal or diary
- Reflective models
- Mind mapping

45

- Supervision
- Journal clubs
- Peer support groups
- Critical incident learning
- CPD portfolios.

Reflective model frameworks are also invaluable for offering a structured continuum for evaluating practice. Each student must explore the tools and use those that complement their own learning style and the choice is likely to vary according to the circumstances of the reflection. See examples of reflective model frameworks below.

Reflective model frameworks

- Gibb's reflective cycle (1988)
- Fish and Twinn (1997)
- Boud et al. (1985)
- Johns (1994)

Methods and Tools of Assessment of the Student

Key aspects and skill areas such as communication, management, therapeutic, professional and reflective skills are incorporated into specific learning outcomes. Educators must develop methods of assessing students that are relevant and appropriate to the placement setting.

The educator can use the following to inform the assessment process:

Methods of assessment

- Observation of a specific task or practical skill undertaken by the student
- Student feedback
- Critical discussion
- Reflection
- Feedback from others – colleagues, patients, team members.

Tools of assessment

- Learning contract as a focus of what needs to be learnt and what has been achieved
- Case studies/presentations to illustrate knowledge and understanding on a specific case or subject
- Portfolio of evidence/placement file to demonstrate collation and synthesis of relevant evidence-based practice

- University criteria – university specific learning outcomes.

A transparent, robust assessment process serves to ensure objectivity and that the student is able to fulfil their potential and thus should reflect attainment of ability, skills and knowledge in practice against pre-determined criteria (Cross et al., 2006).

Students must successfully achieve 1000 assessed hours and pass all their placements in order to graduate. The occupational therapy educators are therefore the gatekeepers to the profession for assessing competence in students' practical skills. It is essential that educators are fully aware of the university's assessment process and confident in making a decision regarding a pass or fail.

Managing Failing and Struggling Students on Placement

There are times when the student's performance on placement does not meet the standard required. This is usually due to two reasons:

- Poor performance due to lack of knowledge and/or skills.
- Poor performance due to ill health and/or personal problems.

It is important that the student is very clear on the expectations for performance on the placement. This should start prior to starting the placement at the preparation sessions in the university, when the university criteria are clarified, at the induction with the educator in the first week of placement where the specific placement expectations are highlighted and continue weekly in the supervision sessions. It is good practice that these are recorded, either as set criteria or in the case of the supervision sessions as a report of each session. Both the student and the educator should sign the supervision records, confirming agreement to the content and its accuracy.

It is important that the student is open with the educator and discusses any health or personal issues that are likely to affect performance on placement. This will allow the educator to take these into consideration where possible.

If the student is not meeting the expectations it is very important that the educator meets with the student as early as possible to highlight his/her concerns and to ask the student if there is anything he/she wishes to share that might be impacting upon his/her performance. Once all parties are clear about the concerns and any mitigating circumstances an action plan can be drafted to assist the student to meet the outcomes. The educator and the student should both have the opportunity to contact the university tutor for further support.

The university tutor will often arrange an early visit to the student and educator so all parties can plan for the rest of the placement. The university tutor should meet with each party separately to ascertain their individual perspectives and then see all parties together to agree an action plan. It is important that the student is clear on expectations. He/she should clarify with the educator throughout the week whether his/her performance is improving and meeting the standard. It is also helpful to the educator if the student justifies his/her decision making as if this is accurate it is a good indicator of clinical reasoning and sound practice. Regular open communication is essential as this informs the other party of the thought processes and decisions being made.

If after the action plans have been put in place and the performance does not improve the student will fail the placement. The student can have the opportunity to continue on the placement, if they wish to and if they are fit to continue, to gain further experience after they have been told they have failed. This will not affect the outcome. However, most students choose to terminate the placement at that point. The student will then have an opportunity to have a repeat placement as a second attempt.

If the student is deemed to be unfit due to ill health/personal problems he/she needs a 'Fit Note' from the GP signing them off work. The terminated placement will then be a deferred placement rather than a failed placement and the student will have an opportunity to repeat the placement as a first attempt, when they are fit.

Evaluating the Experience

It is essential that following each placement both the student and the educator evaluate the experience. This will ensure that the positive elements can be further developed and negative aspects can be addressed for future placements. Table 4.3 indicates methods of evaluating the placement for the educator and student.

Table 4.3 Methods of evaluating the placement

Educator	Student	Both
Report form for student	Evaluation/feedback form to the educator	Reflection
Mentorship	Post-placement workshop/tutorial with university	Peer Evaluation
Audit of feedback from students	Identifying future learning needs	
Feedback from the HEI	Exam board ratification	

Another important aspect of the evaluation stage is for the student to identify the skills and knowledge that they have learnt from placement that they could transfer to future placements/work situations. A useful tool to structure this evaluation could be the use of a SWOT analysis (Strengths, Weaknesses, Opportunities, Threats) of the placement experience, which could aid the student's reflection on the positive and challenging parts of the placement. This could aid the employability of the student when they come to market themselves in their future as they can then identify the transferable skills that they developed through their placement experiences, which can be used in a variety of work settings. There is an example of a SWOT analysis from a placement experience below (Table 4.4) – the focus is on transferable skills so that it is relevant for future employability. This could form an important part of a student's CPD portfolio (see Chapter 9 for more details.)

Table 4.4 SWOT analysis

Strengths (Intrinsic Driving Forces)	**Weaknesses** (Intrinsic Restraining Forces)
Developed skills in writing notes Developed time management skills in a busy acute hospital setting Managed my own caseload Practised peer supervision Developed professional identity in team working.	Difficult to take initiative with a new project Lacked assertiveness skills in MDT meetings Lack of time/priority for supervision.
Opportunities (Extrinsic Driving Forces)	**Threats** (Extrinsic Restraining Forces)
Spent time networking with organisations and promoting occupational therapy in new areas of practice Completed training in Manual Handling and Food Hygiene.	Potential for professional identity to be undermined due to educator being the only OT in the team Staff cuts impacted on number of staff available to learn from.

Conclusion

This chapter has identified the roles and responsibilities of both the educator and the student before and during the placement experience. It has discussed the importance of identifying learning styles and tools that can assist in the process of personal and professional development.

Reflective Questions

1. Following reflection on the roles and responsibilities where do you feel your strengths and areas for development are?

2. Identify a number of reflective tools that you may or may not be familiar with and apply them to a specific learning opportunity. How has this impacted upon your development?

3. Do you know what your personal learning style is? How does this impact upon the effectiveness of your learning?

References

Baird, M. and Winter, J. (2005) 'Reflection, practice and clinical education'. In Rose, M., and Best, D. (eds) *Transforming Practice through Clinical Education, Professional Supervision and Mentoring*. Edinburgh: Elsevier, pp.143–59.

Best, D., Rose, M. and Edwards, H. (2005) 'Learning about learning'. In Rose M., and Best D. (eds) *Transforming Practice through Clinical Education, Professional Supervision and Mentoring*. Edinburgh: Elsevier, pp.121–41.

Biggs, J. (2003) *Teaching for Quality Learning at University*. Maidenhead: Open University Press.

Boud, D., Keogh, R. and Walker, D. (1985) *Reflection: Turning Experience into Learning*. London: Kogan Page.

Brown, L. and Kennedy-Jones, M. (2005) 'Exploring the roles of the clinical educator: Part two: The manager role'. In Rose M., and Best D. (eds) *Transforming Practice through Clinical Education, Professional Supervision and Mentoring*. Edinburgh: Elsevier, pp. 45–86.

College of Occupational Therapists (2006) *APPLE Framework*. London: College of Occupational Therapists.

College of Occupational Therapists (2007) *Professional Standards for Occupational Therapy Practice: Standard Statements*. London: College of Occupational Therapists.

College of Occupational Therapists (2008) *College of Occupational Therapists Pre-registration Education Standards* (3rd edn). London: College of Occupational Therapists.

College of Occupational Therapists (2010) *Code of Ethics and Professional Conduct*. London: College of Occupational Therapists.

Craik, C. (2009) 'Practice Education: skills for students and educators'. In E. Duncan (ed.) *Skills for Practice in Occupational Therapy*. Edinburgh: Churchill Livingstone, pp. 323–35.

Cross, V., Moore, A., Morris., J, Caladine, L., Hilton, R. and Bristow, H. (2006). *The Practice Based Educator: A Reflective Tool for CPD and Accreditation*. Chichester: John Wiley and Sons ltd.

Duke, L .(2004) 'Piecing together the jigsaw: How do practice educators define occupational therapy student competence?' *British Journal of Occupational Therapy*, **67**(5): 201–9.

Field, D.E. (2004) 'Moving from novice to expert – the value of learning in clinical practice: a literature review'. *Nurse Education Today*, **24** (3): 157–9.

Fish, D. and Twinn, S. (1997) *Quality Supervision in the Health Care Professions. Principled Approaches to Practice*. Oxford: Butterworth Heinemann.

Fleming, N. (2010) The VARK Questionnaire. Available at: http://www.vark-learn.com/english/page.asp?p=questionnaire (accessed 26/04/12).

Fry, H., Ketteridge, S. and Marshall, S. (2003) *A Handbook for Teaching and Learning in Higher Education: Enhancing Academic Practice* (2nd edn). Oxon: Routledge Falmer.

Gibbs, G. (1988) *Learning by Doing: A Guide to Teaching and Learning Methods*. Oxford: Further Education Unit.

Gopee, N. (2010). *Practice Teaching in Healthcare*. London: Sage Publications.

Healey, J. and Spencer, M. (2008) *Surviving your Placement in Health and Social Care: A Student Handbook*. Maidenhead: Open University Press.

Health Professions Council (2007) *Standards of Proficiency: Occupational Therapists*. London: Health Professions Council.

Health Professions Council (2008) *Your Guide to our Standards for Continuing Professional Development*. London: Health Professions Council.

Health Professions Council (2009) *Guidance on Conduct and Ethics of Students*. London: Health Professions Council.

Holmes, J., Bossers, A., Polatajko, H., Drynan, D., Gallagher, M., O'Sullivan, C., Slade, A., Stier, J., Storr, C. and Denney, J. (2010) '1000 fieldwork hours: analysis of multi-site evidence.' *Canadian Journal of Occupational Therapy*, **77**(3): 135–143.

Honey, P. and Mumford, A. (2000) *The Learning Styles Questionnaire: 80 Item Version*. Maidenhead: Peter Honey Publications.

Hulme, M. and Hulme, R. (2011) 'Learning styles'. In McIntosh, A., Gidman, J. and Mason-Whitehead, E. (eds) *Key Concepts in Healthcare Education*. London: Sage Publications, pp.100–105.

Johns, C. (1994) 'Nuances of reflection.' *Journal of Clinical Nursing*, **3**: 71–75.

Ledgerd, R. (2005) 'Preparing and developing your work as an allied health professional'. In T. Clouston and L. Westcott. (eds) *Working in Health and Social Care: an introduction for allied health professionals*. Edinburgh: Churchill Livingstone, pp. 187–197.

Matheson, R. (2003) 'Promoting the integration of theory and practice by the use of a learning contract'. *International Journal of Therapy and Rehabilitation*, **10** (6): 264–9.

McBurney, H. (2005) 'Assessor role'. In Rose, M., and Best, D. (eds) *Transforming Practice through Clinical Education, Professional Supervision and Mentoring*. Edinburgh: Elsevier. pp. 77–86.

McIntosh, A. (2011) 'Learning environments'. In McIntosh, A., Gidman J. and Mason-Whitehead, E. (eds) *Key Concepts in Healthcare Education*. London: Sage Publications, pp. 95–100.

Morris, J. (2007) 'Factors influencing the quality of student learning on practice placements'. *Learning in Health and Social Care*, **6**(4): 213–9.

Myall, M., Levett-Jones, T. and Lathlean, J. (2008) 'Mentorship in contemporary practice: the experiences of nursing students and practice mentors'. *Journal of Clinical Nursing* **17** (14): 1834–42.

Neugebauer, J. and Evans-Brain, J.E. (2009) *Making the Most of your Placement*. London: Sage Publications.

The Quality Assurance Agency for Higher Education (2008) *The Framework for Higher Education Qualifications in England, Wales and Northern Ireland*. Mansfield: The Quality Assurance Agency for Higher Education.

Tsang, H., Paterson, M. and Packer, T. (2002) 'Self directed learning in fieldwork education with learning contracts'. *British Journal of Therapy and Rehabilitation*, **9**(5): 184–9.

Webb, G., Fawns, R. and Harré, R. (2009) 'Professional identities and communities of practice'. In Delaney, C. and Molloy, E. (eds) *Clinical Education in the Health Professions*. Sydney: Churchill Livingstone.

Whitcombe, S.W. (2001) 'Using learning contracts in fieldwork education: the views of occupational therapy students and those responsible for their supervision'. *British Journal of Occupational Therapy*, **64** (11): 552–7.

Yueng, E., Jones, A. and Webb, C. (2001) 'The use of learning contracts'. In D. Kember (ed.) *Reflective Teaching and Learning in the Health Professions*. Oxford: Blackwell Publishing, pp. 68–83.

51

Chapter 5
The Occupational Therapy Problem Solving Process on Placement

This chapter is divided into four sections, to replicate the problem-solving process:

- Assessment knowledge and skills
- Planning knowledge and skills
- Intervention knowledge and skills
- Evaluation knowledge and skills

Section 1:
Assessment Knowledge and Skills on Placement

Tracey Polglase and Rachel Treseder

Knowledge and skills relating to assessment form an essential component for occupational therapy students throughout all of their placements. Undertaking an effective assessment requires a unique set of core skills and principles that are transferable across all settings that the student will experience. This section will explore some of these core skills and principles as well as looking at specific tools that may be used to undertake assessments. Four case studies will be used with specific examples of assessments to illustrate their use in a variety of practice settings.

Introduction to Assessment

The aim of assessment is to gather a broad baseline of information about the service user in order to plan intervention collaboratively with them. This baseline of information can then be used at the evaluation stage of the occupational therapy process in order to measure the effectiveness of the intervention. Assessment provides an opportunity for the student and the service user to explore a wide range of issues that will inform the whole occupational therapy process (Duncan, 2011).

Referral Process

In order to start the assessment process a referral needs to be received. Depending on the practice setting there are a number of different referral processes.

Blanket referral

All service users are expected to be seen, e.g. on a ward all service users that are admitted will be referred, there may or may not be a written referral. In this situation the student will be expected to visit the setting on a daily basis to check on new admissions and whether they are suitable for occupational therapy.

Individual referral

Only service users specifically considered to need an occupational therapy assessment will be referred. This is usually via a referral card, letter, telephone or electronic request. The student will need to process the referral according to the policy and procedure of the department and so will need to ensure that they have a full understanding of what this is.

Self referral

A service user or their family/friends can make a referral. This is often seen in social services. The referral often is received by the duty officer – the student may take on this role during their placement.

Information that should be present on the referral

- Personal Details of service user: i.e. name, address, contact telephone number (if not an in-patient), date of birth.
- Reason for referral
- Referrer's name
- Date of referral
- Any other relevant information.

Irrespective of the mode of referral, the service user should be informed and consent given for the referral being made.

Information Gathering

Once a referral has been made it is important for the student to gather essential information. Some of this information may be gathered prior to seeing the service user.

Where to gather information?

Patient's medical notes

Prior to seeing the service user it is valuable for the student to review the medical notes (if available). Key useful information is:

- Past medical/psychiatric history. What conditions they have, how long they have had them, previous hospital admissions, any surgery or treatment.
- Presenting condition. Current reason for admission to hospital or referral to service, present health and functional status.
- Social history. Where they live, who with and social support -informal and formal.

Relatives/friends

Relatives and friends can give valuable information in relation to how the service user has been functioning. It is important to note that relatives and friends should only be contacted after consent to do this has been sought from the service user. If the service user does not have capacity (as assessed by a formal capacity assessment) staff/student need to act in the service user's best interest which could include taking account of information from relatives/friends.

Other professionals

Other professionals can give information on the assessment outcomes and progress they have observed. The student will be expected to liaise with all relevant professionals in order to gather a wide range of information. The service user should be informed that the information and assessment finding will be shared with other members in the team.

Observation

The student can also gather information via observation. This may be done informally prior to seeing the service user, e.g. observing them on the ward or formally during the assessment process. Observable information may support or contradict information being verbally given by the service user, e.g. when asked if the service user is in pain during a specific movement, the service user may say no, but on movement, flinch and restrict the range (contradictory) or may move freely (supporting the statement).

Principles of Assessment

Once sufficient information is gathered about the service user, the student can begin the formal assessment. The following information is important for the student to consider in planning the assessment:

Planning the assessment

- Ensure familiarity with the assessment tool and know how to conduct it.
- Ensure all equipment needed for the assessment is available.

- Book a suitable room to undertake the assessment or make an appointment if the service user is in the community.
- Ensure directions to the property have been confirmed and arrive on time.
- Gather information on the service user prior to the assessment. Research the conditions if unfamiliar with them.

Professional practice

- Introduce self to the service user and inform them about the OT role.
- Obtain consent prior to any intervention.
- Maintain Continuing Professional Development (CPD) in order to practice within the evidence-based practice framework.
- Practice using a client-centred approach.
- Assessment should be holistic considering the service user, their occupations, the environment and the task.
- Teamwork is essential for effective practice. Share information as required.

Types of Assessment

The student may experience a wide range of types of assessments throughout their placement experiences. These tend to fall into five key categories as indicated below.

Shared assessment

This is a standardised process that involves all professionals working collaboratively with the service user. There is one set of notes held centrally. Examples of these include the Single Assessment Process (England) (DoH, 2001), the Unified Assessment (Wales) (WAG, 2003) and the Care Programme Approach (DoH, 1990) for people with mental illness. When working in this way it is important for the professionals/students to have a clear understanding of their own, and others' roles in order to provide the best service (Wilding, 2010).

Initial assessment

The initial assessment is one of the most important assessments that should take place. It is the first contact that the student and service user have with each other and where the therapeutic relationship is established. This assessment involves assimilating the information that has previously been gathered with the information being elicited in the initial interview. The initial interview can be conducted formally completing an assessment document, or informally without documenting information at that point. Both methods are equally valuable; the method adopted will depend on the culture of the department, therapist choice and service user presentation. Full documentation of all assessments should be recorded irrespective of the method of assessment used.

Due to the clinical reasoning and planning that is required during and after the assessment it is essential that it is conducted by a qualified member of staff or a student under the direction of an occupational therapist.

Specific assessments

Following the outcome of the initial assessment the student will decide upon what further assessments need to be completed. The student's degree of autonomy in this process will be dependent on the level of placement, e.g. students on their first placement will be assisted by the educator to undertake this task whereas students in their final placement will be expected to undertake this independently. These assessments will be conducted to ascertain the service user's performance in specific tasks, e.g. functional activities of daily living, hand function, cognitive processing, anxiety levels during specific activities, etc.

The specific assessment results will be combined to produce a holistic picture of the strengths and needs of the individual. The specific assessments can be a combination of standardised and non-standardised assessments. Standardised assessments are those that have been rigorously tested under research conditions to guarantee reliable and valid results. Non-standardised assessments are often designed by the individual departments but have not been through the process of testing for reliability and validity. Service users are often assessed using a combination of the two. Tables 5.1 and 5.2. highlight the advantages and disadvantages of standardised and non-standardised assessments.

Table 5.1 Advantages and disadvantages of standardised assessments

Advantages of standardised assessments	Disadvantages of standardised assessments
Reliable and valid test results	Staff need formal training
Clear guideline on how to conduct assessment	Expensive to purchase
Specific client group stipulated	Some assessments are very time consuming to administer
Some assessments allow for discrete sections to be administered, rather than the whole assessment, thereby overcoming the time consuming disadvantage	Assessment may not be suitable for some service users from different cultures, countries, etc.
Some assessments can be repeated to reliably indicate change	Assessment instructions cannot be changed to aid clarification for the service user. Some assessments have restricted time periods before they can be re-administered, e.g. assessment cannot be re-administered within a 2-month period

Table 5.2 Advantages and disadvantages of non-standardised assessments

Advantages of non-standardised assessments	Disadvantages of non-standardised assessments
Can be conducted informally which can be less stressful	Has the potential for less reliable assessment results
Service users may not feel like they are being assessed	There may be no guidelines on administration therefore different people may administer the assessment differently
No/limited cost implication	

Table 5.3 below lists a range of standardised and non-standardised tests commonly used for different service user groups.

Progress assessments

In a setting where there is a set programme, e.g. 12 weeks, a progress assessment may be undertaken at a specific point, e.g. 6 weeks/half way point. A range of assessments can be repeated in order to review the progress. This is useful for the student as it may indicate whether the service user is progressing as expected or if modifications need to be made. It is also useful for the service user to review his/her own progress as a motivational tool. This can be further supported with video evidence of the service user's presentation at the start of the process and at the specific point of re-assessment. Over a period of time memory of initial presentation fades so video evidence is very useful for both the therapist and the service user. If the programme is long the progress assessment results can be sent to the referrer to indicate how the service user is progressing.

Final Assessment

This will ultimately be an evaluation/outcome measure (also see Section 4, p.94) conducted at the end of the programme in a similar way to the progress assessment. The student should send the referrer the results of this, any further recommendations and a letter confirming that the occupational therapy input is complete.

Commonly Used Assessments

Whilst on placement the student is likely to see and use a wide range of standardised and non-standardised assessments. Table 5.3 lists commonly used assessments for different service user groups.

Table 5.3 Commonly used assessments

Standardised assessment	Non-standardised assessments
Children	**Children**
Movement ABC (Henderson et al., 2007)	Handwriting
Beery-Buktenica Developmental Test of Visual–Motor Integration (Beery et al., 2010)	Hand function
	Play
Detailed Assessment of Speed of Handwriting (DASH) (Barnett et al., 2010)	Self care
Paediatric Evaluation of Disability Inventory (PEDI) (Haley et al., 1992)	Co-ordination assessments
	Wheelchair assessments
Test of playfulness (Bundy, 1997)	Home and school questionnaires
PEGS Paediatric Efficacy and Goal Setting (Missiuna et al., 2004)	
People with a Learning Disability	**People with a Learning Disability**
Assessment of Motor Process Skills (AMPS) (Fisher, 2006)	Activities of Daily Living (personal/domestic/instrumental)
Canadian Occupational Performance Measure (COPM) (Law et al., 2005)	Transfers
	Leisure activities
Model of Human Occupation Screening Tool (Forsyth and Kielhofner, 2011)	Wheelchair assessments
	Environmental/home assessment
Adults	**Adults**
General/Functional	**General/Functional**
Functional Independence Measure/Functional Assessment Measure (FIM/ FAM) (Wright, 2011)	Activities of Daily Living (personal/ domestic/instrumental)
Barthel Index (Shah et al., 1989)	Transfers
Model of Human Occupation Screening Tool Version 2.0 (MOHOST) (Parkinson et al., 2006)	Leisure activities
	Wheelchair assessments
Westmead Home Safety Assessment (Clemson, 1997)	Environmental/home assessment

Adults (cont.)	Adults (cont.)
Psychological/Cognitive	**Psychological/Cognitive**
Hospital Anxiety and Depression Scale (HADS) (Snaith and Zigmond, 1994)	Kim's Game
Becks Depression Inventory (BDI-II) (Beck et al., 1996)	Functional assessments
Clifton Assessment Procedure for the Elderly (CAPE) (Pattie and Gillerad, 1979)	Mental State Examination (Trzepacz and Baker, 1993)
Middlesex Elderly Assessment Mental State (MEAMS) (Golding, 1989)	
Mini Mental State Examination (MMSE) (Folstein et al., 1975)	
Large Allen's Cognitive Level Screen (LACLS– 5) (Allen et al., 2007)	
Neurological	**Neurological**
Rivermead Perceptual Assessment Battery (1991) (Whiting et al., 1991)	Sensory testing
Chessington Occupational Therapy Neurological Assessment Battery (COTNAB) (Tyerman et al., 1986)	Stereognosis sensory bag
Structured Observation Test of Function – (SOTOF) (Laver and Powell, 1995)	
Productivity	**Productivity**
Volitional questionnaire (VQ) (De las Heras et al., 2007)	Work place assessment
Leisure	**Leisure**
Volitional questionnaire (VQ) (De las Heras et al., 2007)	Interest checklist

Case Studies to Illustrate Application of Assessments on Placement

Below are four case studies to illustrate the application of a range of assessments on placement (Tables 5.4, 5.5, 5.6, and 5.7).

Table 5.4 Case study 1: Adult male with a spinal injury

Background
Tim is 23 years old. He lives with his fiancée (Mandy) and 2-year-old son (Jordan) in a rented, two storey house. Tim works as a roofer and Mandy works part time as a ward receptionist.

Diagnosis + Presentation
Tim fell from the roof, 30 feet onto the ground, and sustained a complete spinal injury at C6. He has been in the regional spinal injury unit for two weeks after spending one month on the acute neurology ward of the local hospital. In addition to the spinal injury Tim also sustained a fractured right femur, deep laceration to right forearm and concussion. He is struggling to come to terms with his injuries and has been diagnosed with depression; this is impacting upon his motivation to participate in therapy.

Choice of OT Assessments + Justification	
Assessment	**Justification**
Initial Interview	To gain information from the service user's perspective. Establish baseline
Hand Function Assessment	Certain function can be achieved with splints, etc.
Becks Depression Inventory (Beck *et al.*, 1996)	Depression has been highlighted
Powered Wheelchair and Cushion Assessment	Tim will be unable to walk or relieve pressure, therefore a suitable wheelchair and cushion is required
Home Assessment with Social Services Occupational Therapist	Service user plans to return home. Home needs major adaptations or transfer to meet Tim's needs
Interest Checklist	To ascertain occupations/hobbies that are important to Tim
Work/Training Assessment	Late assessment to ascertain Tim's skills for future employment/education opportunities

Description of Assessment and Application
Initial Interview
The initial interview schedule would follow the format of the model chosen. It is important to conduct the assessment to incorporate a holistic approach. As Tim is low in mood this assessment needs to be conducted sensitively and due to his poor motivation it is important to work slowly with him to build up trust and rapport. The interview may need to be conducted over a number of sessions in an informal manner. Tim may be feeling like he has very little control over anything so giving him elements of choice will assist him in regaining some control. At this stage it is important to ascertain Tim's priorities.
Hand Function Assessment
At this level of injury Tim will be able to use a tenodesis grip and this can be enhanced by the use of a dynamic splint. Once this has been established further assessments can be undertaken using the splint e.g. feeding, cleaning teeth, writing, keyboard use, etc.
Beck Depression Inventory (BDI-II) (Beck et al., 1996)
The BDI-II is a self-administered questionnaire of 21 questions with four multiple choice answers. Each element is scored 0–3. Overall scores of 0–13 = minimal depression; 14–19 = mild depression; 20–28 = moderate depression and 29–63 = severe depression. This can be given to Tim to complete independently in his own time. He will need to be competently using his splint to be able to write. Alternatively the assessment could be conducted in an interview format with the student reading out the questions and answers, Tim responding and the student completing the form.
Powered Wheelchair and Cushion
A suitable indoor/outdoor powered chair will be required, together with a pressure relieving cushion. The key function will be to regain mobility and facilitate engagement in occupations. There is a standardised wheelchair and pressure cushion form to complete from the local wheelchair service. (Basic information includes height, weight, limb measurements, posture, diagnosis, function and functional limitations, type of controls, etc.) Pressure relieving cushions are designed to maintain skin integrity by redistributing pressure over a wider area. They are constructed using air, gel, foam or a combination.
Home Assessment
The student needs to be aware that this assessment is likely to be conducted with the OT from the spinal injury unit and the local social services OT. There may be several assessments conducted due to the complexity of need.

The initial assessment of the property can be conducted without Tim. If it is decided that Tim's property is suitable, certain adaptations will be required, e.g. level access to the property and throughout the ground floor, door widths to accommodate the wheelchair, all facilities on ground floor, e.g. bedroom, kitchen, lounge, bathroom and toilet. This may require a Disabled Facilities Grant (DFG), which the Social Services Occupational Therapist will be responsible for. If the property is not suitable for adaptation the other option is re-housing to an adapted property.

Interest Checklist

It is important for the student to ascertain occupations and hobbies that are important to Tim. These can then be incorporated into the intervention programme, e.g. computer games to facilitate improved hand function.

Work/Training Assessment

This will be conducted late in the rehabilitation process. Tim will be unable to return to his previous employment so an assessment of his abilities and limitations can be undertaken alongside the Disability Employment Advisor (DEA) within the job centre to consider suitable future training/ employment.

Table 5.5 Case study 2: Older adult female with multiple pathology

Background
Mrs Jones is 83 years old. She lives alone in a terraced property with bedroom and bathroom upstairs. She has community alarm and a small package of care. Carers call on Wednesday to do the shopping and Friday to assist with showering. Family manage Mrs Jones' finances.

Diagnosis + Presentation
Mrs Jones was admitted into hospital following a fall at home when she got up at night to use the toilet. On admission she was cold, confused and complaining of pain in her hip and back. She has stated that she is anxious about falling again and injuring herself. On examination it has been concluded that Mrs Jones has no fractures but severe bruising. The fall was caused by poor footwear and tripping over the corner of a rug. There is a past medical history of mild dementia, transient ischaemic attacks (TIAs) (x2), osteoarthritis of the hips and right knee and non-insulin dependent diabetes mellitus (NIDDM).

Choice of Assessments + Justification	
Assessment	**Justification**
Initial Interview	To gain information from the service user's perspective. Establish baseline
Pain Analogue Scale	Pain has been highlighted as a problem
Personal Care Assessment	Service user was undertaking this task prior to admission and wishes to resume this
Kitchen Assessment	Service user was undertaking this task prior to admission and wishes to resume this
Mini Mental State Examination (Folstein et al., 1975)	Some confusion has been highlighted
Westmead Home Safety Assessment (Clemson, 1997)	Service user has fallen and has a fear of further falls
Home Assessment	Hazards at home highlighted. Service user plans to return home
Interest Checklist	To ascertain occupations/hobbies that are important to Mrs Jones

Description of Assessment and Application

Initial Interview

An initial interview following the model format can be conducted to ascertain background information and the service user's perspective. It is important that this assessment is conducted in a quiet environment without distractions to ensure Mrs Jones can perform at her optimum.

Pain Analogue Scale

This is a simple test to ascertain Mrs Jones' subjective pain levels. The scale is 1–10 with 1 = no pain and 10 = excruciating pain. Mrs Jones is asked to rate her pain during certain activities. Pain can seriously impact upon function and concentration so managing the pain is very important.

Personal Care Assessment

This can be undertaken on the ward at a suitable time, e.g. after breakfast. For best results the assessment should be conducted following the process Mrs Jones normally follows. It is important to specifically record what the person can manage independently and what they require assistance with. The assessment should consider functional performance, cognition, sequencing and safety recognition.

Kitchen/Domestic Assessment

Prior to the assessment it is important for the student to clarify what Mrs Jones does at home and to replicate this. There is no point assessing ability to make a 3-course meal if Mrs Jones only heats a readymade meal in the microwave. It is important to specifically record what the person can manage independently and what they require assistance with. The assessment should consider functional performance, cognition, sequencing and safety recognition.

Mini Mental State Examination (Folstein *et al.*, 1975)

This screening tool is used widely in the UK. There are groups of questions to test areas such as orientation in time and place, memory, attention/concentration, language, comprehension of commands, and spelling and grammar. It is important to ensure Mrs Jones wears her glasses and hearing aid if she needs them. The test should be conducted in a quiet room without distractions to ensure the best outcome. The test is scored out of 30 and if she scores below 23 it is indicative of cognitive impairment.

Falls

The Westmead Home Safety Assessment (Clemson, 1997) is a 72-point checklist to assess people at home who have fallen or are at risk of falling. It would be conducted by walking Mrs Jones around her home and rating each point as relevant or not, then for the relevant aspects highlighting if they are a hazard or not. Each element is scored and a report completed.

Home Assessment

Following assessments in the hospital it is important to assess Mrs Jones' performance and safety in her home. It is useful to use a checklist for this purpose. A logical method that could be adopted would be to ask Mrs Jones to walk the student through the property, this way her mobility and orientation can be assessed informally, without her feeling as if she is being tested. Environmental issues can also be observed, e.g. flooring, lighting, steps, etc. Functional assessments can be carried out during the process, e.g. making a cup of tea, carrying it to the favourite seating area, transfers etc. Any hazards can be highlighted and solutions discussed over a cup of tea.

Interest Checklist

Often older people's leisure occupations are ignored, but they are the group of people who often have the most time for leisure. It is important to ask Mrs Jones what she does with her time, whether she is content with it and if she would like to experience anything new. This can then be incorporated into the treatment programme.

Table 5.6 Case study 3: Adult male with anxiety and depression

Background
Jeff is 45 years old and recently divorced. He has a stressful job and works a 60-hour week. He lives alone in a self-contained apartment in the city centre and sees his two children, Daniel (15) and Lucy (13) every other weekend.

Diagnosis + Presentation
Jeff has recently started experiencing panic attacks whilst at work which has impacted on his ability to function properly. He is having trouble sleeping and has little appetite. He has also just started smoking again after 15 years. His GP has recently signed him off work with a diagnosis of clinical depression and acute anxiety. He now rarely leaves the house, and his main contact with anyone is his fortnightly meeting with his two children and sister Sarah, who lives approximately 20 miles away.

Choice of Assessments and Justification	
Assessment	**Justification**
Initial Interview using Mental State Examination (Trzepacz and Baker, 1993)	To gain information from the service user's perspective. Establish baseline
Hospital Anxiety and Depression scale (HADS) (Snaith and Zigmond, 1994)	To determine level and differentiation between depression and anxiety
Occupational questionnaire (Smith *et al.*, 1986)	To demonstrate balance of activity prior to ill health and determine Jeff's level of motivation to undertake particular occupations
Home Assessment	Assessment of Jeff in his natural environment will provide a more holistic picture of Jeff and his strengths and needs

Description of Assessment and Application
Initial Interview using Mental State Examination
The structure provided by the mental state examination will allow an exploration of specific areas that will provide insight into Jeff's current state of mind. These domains include: Appearance Attitude Behaviour

Mood and affect

Speech

Thought process

Thought content

Perception

Cognition

Insight and judgement. (Trzepacz and Baker, 1993)

Through discussion with Jeff and observation during this initial assessment, a more holistic picture will be gathered of his current mental state, which will form significant baseline information when planning intervention. It is very important that an optimum therapeutic relationship is established early on in the assessment process. The student will use herself as a therapeutic tool in the occupational therapy process and so needs to establish trust and a good rapport at the outset.

Occupational Questionnaire (Smith et al., 1986)

Based on the Model of Human Occupation this assessment tool is effective in identifying occupational balance and the motivational drive for specific activities. Due to the clear imbalance in occupations in Jeff's life prior to his illness, the occupational questionnaire will be an effective tool to illustrate this. The student will work with Jeff to complete the timetable demonstrating the breakdown of his time on an hourly basis for an average working day. He will then be encouraged to categorise each activity as work, a daily living task, recreation or rest (Creek and Bullock 2008). Following this the student will work with Jeff to rate each activity on a scale of 1–5 for personal causation (how well he thinks he performs it), values (how important it is to him) and interest (how much he enjoys it) (Creek, 2008). This information will allow Jeff and the student in collaboration to identify potential causes of his anxiety, occupational imbalance and setting of realistic therapeutic goals to address this.

Home Assessment

Although Jeff does not have any physical limitations, his home environment is crucial to his health and well-being. The student will be able to gain a more holistic picture of Jeff's current level of functioning through an assessment of his home environment. This will need to ascertain constraints and demands offered by his environment. Assessment information may include consideration of how Jeff functions within his home, accessibility to support, community facilities, etc , what particular roles Jeff has within his home environment, and level of motivation to undertake tasks within his home environment.

Table 5.7 Case study 4: Adolescent female with a learning disability

Background
Sally is 17 years old and has Down's Syndrome. She currently lives with her mother and younger sister in a small terraced house. Her father left home when she was 3 years old and she has regular contact with him twice a month. Sally attended a mainstream school to the age of 16. She developed a good network of friends and functioned well within this environment. She is now moving on to adult services and will be attending college to train in catering. She has also started expressing a desire to move into a group home with her friends. Her mother is not keen on this idea as she feels Sally is not ready for this step yet.

Diagnosis and Presentation
Sally has been referred to the community learning disability team as she has recently been displaying signs of challenging behaviour. She has become verbally aggressive with her mother and sister, which is distressing them. This is noticeably worse when she is due to visit her father. She has a good appetite and appears to comfort eat when she is distressed, and so she is putting on weight. She is also sleeping a lot, and does not want to get up in the mornings.

Choice of Assessments + Justification	
Assessment	**Justification**
Information gathering for transition to adult services and assessment of challenging behaviour	Sally is approaching transition from child to adult services and so it is imperative that the occupational therapist gathers relevant information from children's services to enable smooth transition. There are also many potential triggers of Sally's presenting behaviour; although it is not possible to observe all of these, it is important for the therapist to gain a holistic picture of potential triggers and methods of communication used in Sally's social environment
Non-standardised observation of leisure activity	To build therapeutic relationship with Sally, and observe communication skills in a non-threatening environment
Model of Human Occupation Screening Tool (MOHOST) (Parkinson et al. 2006)	A holistic initial standardised assessment which will present a comprehensive picture of existing skills to be transferred to new environments

Description of Assessment and Application

Information Gathering

If possible the student will need to gather information from various sources to gain a holistic picture of Sally, particularly in relation to her challenging behaviour. These will include Sally's family and her teacher at school in order to identify potential patterns of stress within Sally's social environment. Most importantly the student should gain consent and gather information from Sally herself in order to identify effective methods of communication and potential barriers to these. The student will also need to gather information in relation to transition; these will include the occupational therapist from children's services, the transition plan that should have been written by the headteacher from Sally's school, and professionals from other agencies that may have been involved in Sally's care (e.g. speech therapist). This will enable the student to formulate baseline assessment to plan appropriate intervention to enable transition and address the challenging behaviour.

Observation of Leisure Activity

The need to establish Sally's methods of communication can be facilitated by a shared activity; Sally enjoys cooking and so the student meets her at home to prepare a healthy meal with her. (The student will need to ensure adherence to her lone working policy from her workplace, and that her own safety is not compromised.) This gives her the opportunity to establish a working relationship using an activity that she enjoys, whilst observing her skills undertaking a specific task. She is also able to meet her mother and sister, which provides a greater understanding of Sally's social environment.

The Model of Human Occupation Screening Tool (MOHOST) Version 2.0 (Parkinson et al., 2006)

This is a comprehensive assessment that enables the student to identify Sally's current skill base that can be transferred to her new learning environment and identify new skills that need to be learnt (Hurst, 2009). From this screening tool the student is able to formulate her assessment information using the following headings:

Motivation for occupation – appraisal of ability/expectations of success/interest/commitment

Pattern of occupation – routine and adaptability/responsibility and roles

Communication and interaction skills

Process skills

Environment

Motor skills

Conclusion

This section of the chapter has presented the key principles of assessment together with common assessments that the student may experience on placement. These have been applied to specific case scenarios that have covered the life cycle and a range of different conditions.

Reflective Questions

1. What range of assessments have you observed/practiced during your placements?

2. What skills have you developed to enable you to assess more effectively?

3. What do you think you need more experience in to assess more effectively? How might you get this experience?

4. How might you transfer your assessment skills from one placement to the next?

References

Allen, C.K., Austin, S.L., David, S.K., Earhart, C.A., McCraith, D.B., and Riska-Williams, L. (2007) *Large Allen Cognitive Level Screen – 5 (LACLS – 5)*, Camarillo, CA: ACLS and LACLS Committee.

Barnett, A., Henderson, S.E., Scheib, and B., Schulz, J. (2010) *Detailed Assessment of Speed of Handwriting (DASH 17+)*. Pearson Assessment: Psychcorp UK. Available at, http://www.psychcorp.co.uk (accessed 26/04/12).

Beck, A.T., Steer, R.A., Ball, R., and Ranieri, W. (1996) 'Comparison of Beck Depression Inventories -IA and -II in Psychiatric Outpatients'. *Journal of Personality Assessment*, **67**(3): 588–97.

Beery, N.A., Buktenica, N.A., and Beery, K.E., (2010) *Beery-Buktenica Developmental Test of Visual-Motor Integration*, Sixth Edition. Minneapolis: Pearson.

Bundy, A.C. (1997), 'Play and playfulness: What to look for'. In L.D. Parham and L.S. Fazio (eds), *Play in Occupational Therapy for Children* (pp. 52–66). St. Louis: Mosby.

Clemson, L. (1997) *Home Fall Hazards: A guide to identifying fall hazards in the homes of elderly people and an accompaniment to the assessment tool, the Westmead Home Safety Assessment*. West Brunswick, Victoria, Australia: Coordinates Publication.

Creek, J. and Bullock, A. (2008) 'Assessment and outcome measures.' In J. Creek and L. Lougher (eds) *Occupational Therapy and Mental Health* (4th edn). London: Churchill Livingstone.

De las Heras, C.G., Geist, R., Kielhofner, G., and Li, Y. (2007) *Volitional Questionnaire*. 4th edition. Available at http://www.uic.edu/depts/moho/assess/vq.html (accessed 26/04/12).

Department of Health (DoH) (1990) *The Care Programme Approach for People with a Severe Mental Illness Referred to the Specialist Psychiatric Services*. London: The Stationery Office.

Department of Health (DoH) (2001) *The National Service Framework for Older People*. London: The Stationery Office.

Duncan, E.A.S. (2011) 'Skills and processes in occupational therapy', in E.A.S Duncan (ed.) *Foundations for Practice in Occupational Therapy*. (5th Edition). Edinburgh: Elsevier, pp. 33–42.

Fisher, A.G. (2006) AMPS *Assessment of Motor and Process Skills Volume 1: development, standardization, and administration manual*, (6th Edition). Colorado, USA: Three Star Press Inc

Folstein, M.F., and Folstein, S.E., McHugh, P.R. (1975) '"Mini-mental state": A practical method for grading the cognitive state of patients for the clinician'. *Journal of Psychiatric Research*, **12**(3): 189–98.

Forsyth, K. and Kielhofner, G. (2011) 'The model of human occupation: embracing the complexity of occupation by integrating theory into practice and practice into theory'. In E.A.S. Duncan (ed.) *Foundations for Practice in Occupational Therapy* (5th Edition). Edinburgh: Elsevier, pp. 51–80.

Golding, E. (1989) *Middlesex Elderly Assessment of Mental State (MEAMS)*. Essex: Pearson Education Ltd.

Haley, S.M., Coster, W.J., Ludlow, L.H., Haltiwanger, J.T. and Andrellos, P.J. (1992) *Paediatric Evaluation of Disability Inventory*. San Antonio: Pearson Education Inc.

Henderson, S.E., Sugden, D.A., and Barnett, A.L. (2007) *Movement Assessment Battery for Children – 2 (Movement ABC – 2) Examiners Manual.* London: Harcourt Assessment.

Hurst, J. (2009) 'The challenges of maintaining occupation at times of transition' in J. Goodman, J. Hurst and C. Locke (eds) *Occupational Therapy for People with Learning Disabilities, A Practical Guide*. London: Churchill Livingstone, pp. 149–160.

Laver, A.J., and Powell, G. (1995) *The Structured Observational Test of Function*. Windsor: NFER-Nelson.

Law, M., Baptiste, S., Carswell, A., McColl, M.A., Polatajko, H., and Pollock, N. (2005) *Canadian Occupational Performance Measure*, 4th Edition. Ottawa: CAOT Publications ACE.

Missiuna, C., Pollock, N., and Law, M. (2004) *Perceived Efficacy and Goal Setting System (PEGS)*. San Antonio: Psychological Corporation.

Parkinson, S., Forsyth, K. and Kielhofner, G. (2006) *Model of Human Occupation Screening Tool: Version 2.0.* Available at http://www.uic.edu/depts/moho/assess/mohost.html (accessed 26/04/12).

Pattie, A.H. and Gillerad, C. (1979) *Clifton Assessment Procedures for the Elderly (CAPE).* London: Hodder and Stoughton.

Shah, S., Vanclay, F. and Cooper, B. (1989) 'Improving the sensitivity of the Barthel Index for Stroke Rehabilitation'. *Journal of Clinical Epidemiology* **42**: 703–709.

Smith, N.R., Kielhofner, G., and Watts, J.H. (1986) 'The relationships between volition, activity pattern, and life satisfaction in the elderly'. *American Journal of Occupational Therapy,* **40**: 278–283.

Snaith, R.P. and Zigmond, A.S. (1994) *The Hospital Anxiety and Depression Scale*. Windsor: NFER Nelson.

Tyerman, R.T., Tyerman, A., Howard, P., and Hadfield, C. (1986) *Chessington Occupational Therapy Neurological Assessment Battery (COTNAB)*. Nottingham Rehabilitation.

Trzepacz, P.T., and Baker R.W. (1993) *The Psychiatric Mental Status Examination*. Oxford, U.K.: Oxford University Press.

Welsh Assembly Government (2003) *The Strategy for Older People in Wales*. Cardiff: Welsh Assembly Government.

Whiting, S., Lincoln, N., Cockburn, J. and Bhavnani, G. (1991) *Rivermead Perceptual Assessment Battery*. Windsor: NFER-Nelson.

Wilding, C. (2010) 'Defining occupational therapy' in M. Curtin, M. Molineux and J. Supyk-Mellson. *Occupational Therapy and Physical Dysfunction: Enabling Occupation*. Edinburgh: Elsevier pp. 3–16.

Wright, J. (2000). *The Functional Assessment Measure* The Centre for Outcome Measurement in Brain Injury. Available at http://www.tbims.org/combi/FAM (accessed 26/04/12).

Section 2:
Planning Knowledge and Skills on Placement

Tracey Polglase and Rachel Treseder

Introduction to Planning Knowledge and Skills

Planning is considered to be the second phase of the problem solving process and follows on from the assessment stage for the service user. This section will present key issues that students need to consider when planning for the service user and considerations for their professional planning issues on placement.

Within occupational therapy there is an expectation for client-centred holistic practice to take place. In order for this to be possible the whole problem solving process needs to be followed and the student needs to ensure the service user is an active participant and centrally focused at all stages. Latham (2004) and Locke and Latham (2002) have shown that active participation of the service user in planning leads to increased motivation and this has a positive impact on skill development. It is important for the student to be aware that the planning stage is often more inherently integrated into the whole process so that it is not always evidenced as clearly as the other stages. The student may therefore need to ask more questions in relation to this to ensure understanding and accuracy of assumptions.

Planning for the Service User

The planning stage should be considered the glue between assessment and intervention.

The findings from the assessment undertaken by the student may highlight three key elements:

- Strengths: Aspects the service user is able to achieve or are of benefit, e.g. independently mobile, well motivated, ground floor accommodation, etc.

- Limitations: Aspects the service user is unable to achieve or are restrictive, e.g. unable to transfer independently, poor short term memory, no family support.

- Needs: Aspects the service user wants to improve or address, e.g. increase mobility, use memory aids, access property safely.

As can be seen these elements may be physical, psychological or social in nature. Students often confuse 'limitations' with 'needs'. As illustrated they are distinctly different. 'Limitations' can be considered negative in context, but 'Needs' focus on addressing issues in order to improve.

A tip to avoid confusing them is to use the terms as precursors when listing them, e.g.

Mrs X's limitations are............

Mrs X's needs to..........

Aims/goals and objectives

Probably the most common way to record the planning stage is to use Aims/Goal and Objectives. It is important to define these terms and to use them correctly:

- Aims/goals are the targets. They may be vague and woolly (bit like a sheep!). They do not indicate how the target is achieved, just what it is.
- Objectives are the means to reach the target. They should be occupationally focused, written for the service user and SMART.

Park (2009) indicates the meaning of SMART:

S = Specific

M = Measurable

A = Attainable

R = Realistic

T = Timely

Students need to ensure all of these elements are evident in the objective for it to be effective. Occupational therapy students need to be skilled and competent in writing SMART occupationally focused objectives with service users. If they are vague they will lack direction and consequently lead to poor achievement.

Aims/goals and objectives are usually divided into short term, intermediate term and long term (Creek and Bullock, 2008), but for the purpose of this text the long term and short term will only be used as these are what are most commonly seen on placement. By dividing them in this way it indicates the grading of the process and the prioritisation system. When planning a programme using a graded approach the student should break down the activity to its component parts (task/activity analysis) and then decide how to grade the activity progressively. The student may also adapt the activity to match the service user's ability. The skill is in presenting an activity that is achievable at the same time as being challenging. An activity that is not achievable could have a negative impact upon the services user's motivation and self esteem. This would be particularly relevant when in a placement setting with service users who have mental health problems or are lacking in confidence. An activity that is not challenging could reduce the speed of recovery for the service user. This could be seen in an orthopaedic or neurological rehabilitation setting where lack of challenge will impact markedly upon recovery. It must also be remembered that grading is not a one way process, e.g. students in placement settings seeing service users with degenerating conditions or those with a terminal illness may need to grade the activity to make it easier to achieve as the service user deteriorates.

In using this system the process can be illustrated using a pyramid structure, see Figure 5.1.

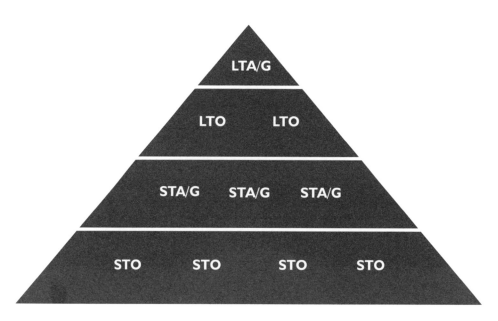

Figure 5.1 Pyramid of aims/goals and objectives

The top of the pyramid is the long term aim/goal (LTA/G). This is the ultimate target. In order to achieve this there should be a number of long term objectives (LTO) indicating the activities required to achieve the long term aim/goal. Below this are the short term aims/goals (STA/G). They are the targets to be achieved first. For each short term aim/goal there should be a number of short term objectives (STO).

All aims/goals and objectives should be written for the service user, not the therapist/student (Park 2009). A common error is to write the objectives as a list of activities for the student to undertake. See examples below of the correct way (✔☺) and incorrect way (✘☹) to write an objective.

✔☺ Mrs X to independently and safely use the toilet, fitted with the raised toilet seat, by the end of week 2.

✘☹ To provide Mrs X with a raised toilet seat for her toilet.

As can be seen, the first example is clearly service user focused and is written to incorporate all elements of SMART. The second example is merely a prompt for the student to provide a piece of equipment. It is also not SMART.

Goal planning meetings

These are often seen in rehabilitation placement settings. A regular meeting takes place (e.g. monthly) to set and review the goals of each service user. The meeting is attended by all the staff involved in the care (and part or all of the meeting may be open to the service user and his/her relatives/carers for their input). The goals are set for each element of care. This is agreed between the service user and the staff. This type of meeting is considered invaluable as it encourages collaborative working thereby avoiding duplication and facilitating interventions that are complementary.

It is essential that the service user is involved in this process as this will ensure he/she is aware of the goals and this will encourage greater compliance and motivation to achieve them (Latham 2004).

Care Programme Approach (CPA) (DoH, 1990)

The CPA is a whole process approach that is predominantly used in mental health placement settings. It is included in the planning section as it is ultimately an inter-professional approach to the planning of care and therapy. There is one set of paperwork that records the assessments undertaken, their results and the plan of action across professional and agency boundaries. Specific intervals for re-assessment and review are recorded and take place. There are two distinct levels of care, 'standard' and 'enhanced' (DoH 1996). Students must ensure they understand and accurately follow the procedures when using this approach.

Tools to assist in the planning process

Although tools such as outcome measures are ultimately used as part of the evaluation process, they are also used to assist in goal setting e.g. *Canadian Occupational Performance Measure* (COPM) (Law et al., 2005), *Goal Attainment Scaling* (GAS) (Kiresuk and Sherman, 1968) and *Perceived Efficacy and Goal Setting System* (PEGS) (Missiuna et al., 2004).

When undertaking any planning it is important to incorporate an element of flexibility to ensure the programme can adapt to changing circumstances.

Planning for the Professional

In addition to the planning specifically related to the service user the therapist/student also needs to undertake planning from a professional perspective. This will include the following:

Preparation work prior to seeing a service user.

Once a referral has been received the student should check any relevant records, e.g. previous OT notes, medical records, nurses' Kardex, etc. to clarify details. It may also be necessary to contact the referrer for more information. The student might also need to undertake further reading/research to clarify issues regarding the condition, presentation, prognosis, potential intervention etc. as this will inform his/her practice.

Organisation of self

In order to see the service user the student needs to arrange an appointment. This may be:

1. A visit to the ward to see them if they are in hospital (e.g. physical/mental health in-patient placement settings).

2. Contacting them at home by letter or phone to make an appointment to visit them (e.g. social services, community rehabilitation placement settings).

3. Contacting them at home by letter or phone to invite them to come into the OT department as an out-patient (e.g. clinic/out-patient placement settings).

When seeing the service user it is important that the student has all essential documentation, information and equipment with him/her.

Prioritising

Therapists and students will carry a caseload and they will need to decide on the order they plan to see the service users. The simplest method of doing this is to see them in date order of referral, however there are often variables that impact upon this decision making process, e.g. health of the service user, if an in-patient planned date of discharge and location, complexity of involvement, etc. The student should follow the departmental protocol.

Liaising with other staff

The value of collaborative working is well documented and stipulated in COT (2010) and HPC (2008). Within the planning context it is important that information is shared between the parties. N.B. Information should only be shared with the consent of the service user.

In a rehabilitation placement setting it is also essential that staff liaise with each other regarding when they are seeing service users. This may be organised with a timetable. There should be consideration of the need for rest periods between certain sessions or one may need to be done before the other.

Records

It is essential that the planning is clearly recorded by the student in the service user's notes. This should indicate the aims, objectives and priority of achieving these. The stage the service user has achieved should be clearly evident, together with the plan for the next session (Bowman and Mogensen 2010). The College of Occupational Therapists (COT) (2010) and the Health Professions Council (HPC) (2008) indicate the therapist's/student's duty in relation to record keeping. A commonly used structured system for recording notes is to use the SOAP acronym to record the data gathered:

- Subjective
- Objective
- Assessment
- Plan

The information is recorded in this format each time the service user is seen within the treatment programme.

Conclusion

An effective planning process is essential in order for the student to transfer the information gathered in the assessment stage into a service user focused intervention programme. There are different methods used but the most important consideration should be that the planning is flexible to meet changing needs and is negotiated with the service user. This section has presented the planning considerations for the service user and the personal planning considerations that the student needs to be aware of during practice.

Reflective Questions

1. Reflecting on your practice placements so far, how client-centred are you? Where can you improve?

2. Use a tool to assist your planning process on placement, then analyse how it has impacted upon your practice.

3. How might you transfer your planning skills from one placement to another?

References

Bowman, J. and Mogensen, L.L. (2010) 'Writing occupationally focused goals' in M. Curtin, M. Molineux and J. Supyk-Mellson *Occupational Therapy and Physical Dysfunction: Enabling Occupation*. Edinburgh: Elsevier, pp. 95–109.

College of Occupational Therapists (2010) *Code of Ethics and Professional Conduct*. London: College of Occupational Therapists.

Creek, J. and Bullock, A. (2008) 'Planning and implementation' in J. Creek and L. Lougher, *Occupational Therapy and Mental Health* (4th Edition). Edinburgh: Elsevier, pp.109–130.

Department of Health (DoH) (1990) *The Care Programme Approach for People with a Severe Mental Illness Referred to the Specialist Psychiatric Services*. London: The Stationery Office.

Department of Health (DoH) (1996) *Effective Co-ordination in Mental Health Services: Modernising the Care Programme Approach*. London: The Stationery Office.

Health Professions Council (2008) *Standards of Conduct, Performance and Ethics*. London: Health Professions Council.

Kiresuk, T.J. and Sherman, R.E. (1968) 'Goal attainment scaling: A general method for evaluating comprehensive community mental health programmes'. *Community Mental Health Journal*, 4(6): 443–453.

Latham, G.P. (2004) 'The motivational benefits of goal setting'. *Academy of Management Executive*, 18(4): 126–129.

Law, M., Baptiste, S., Carswell, A., McColl, M.A., Polatajko, H. and Pollock, N. (2005) *Canadian Occupational Performance Measure*, 4th Edition. Ottawa: CAOT Publications ACE.

Locke, E. A. and Latham, G.P. (2002) 'Building a practically useful theory of goal setting and task motivation'. *American Psychologist*, 57(9): 705–717.

Missiuna, C., Pollock, N. and Law, M. (2004). *Perceived Efficacy and Goal Setting System (PEGS)*. San Antonio: Psychological Corporation.

Park, S. (2009) 'Goal setting in occupational therapy: A client-centred perspective'. In E.A.S. Duncan, *Skills for Practice in Occupational Therapy*. Edinburgh: Elsevier, pp.105–122.

Section 3:
Intervention Knowledge and Skills on Placement

Rachel Treseder and Tracey Polglase

Introduction

Students will inevitably experience a wide range of interventions throughout their placements that are used as part of the occupational therapy process. The diverse range of therapeutic media used will require a set of skills and knowledge that are transferable across different settings, in addition to specialised skills that are learnt in specific settings.

This section of the chapter will address the principles of intervention as part of the occupational therapy process. Four case studies will be used to illustrate types of intervention that students may find on placement and the variety of theoretical approaches that drive the intervention.

Definition

Intervention is the stage of the occupational therapy process that follows assessment and planning and involves putting the 'plan into action' (Creek, 2003). Although many occupational therapy interventions may appear fairly simplistic, it is actually a complex process that requires knowledge and expertise to manage. The main focus of occupational therapy intervention may be largely dictated by the setting that the student is working in, time and resources that are available, but there are certain principles to the intervention stage that are non-negotiable and form part of the philosophy of the profession. It is important that the student has a firm understanding of these principles from the outset.

Principles of Occupational Therapy Intervention

As discussed in earlier chapters, occupational therapy is based on a complex interplay between the person, their environment and their occupations and the relationship between these three components and the health of the individual (Hocking and Ness, 2002). When considering the intervention stage of the therapeutic process, it is even more crucial that all three areas are accounted for.

Occupational focus

The profession of occupational therapy is based upon the principle that we are occupational beings and have an innate need to be occupied. Occupational therapists take this a stage further and highlight the therapeutic value of occupation and the potentially 'transformational power' available 'when the choices and processes are personally meaningful' (Watson and Swartz, 2004, p. 19).

Therefore the student will learn that the intervention stage will involve engaging the service user in activities that are purposeful to them. These activities may be drawn from any aspect of occupation that an individual can engage in, whether that is work, self-care or leisure (Creek, 2003). The student will use their knowledge and skills related to occupation to meet the aims of treatment (see Table 5.8) identified in the planning stage.

Table 5.8 Knowledge and skills about occupation required for effective intervention
(Adapted from Hocking and Ness, 2002, p 14)

Knowledge of Occupation
What is occupation?
Cultural influences on occupation
Why do people engage in occupation?
How is occupation performed and organised?
The characteristics of skilful performance
The temporal aspects of occupation
The subjective experience and personal meaningfulness of occupation
The outcomes of occupation for the individual, the group or society, and the environment
How can occupation be used therapeutically to influence health, and to increase participation or satisfaction with participation?

The intervention skills required for effective intervention related to occupation are analysing, adapting and grading occupation together with using occupation therapeutically. The student will use the above knowledge of occupation in the application of these skills.

Person

Another important aspect for the student to consider is the individual person that they are working with. Sumsion (2006) has written extensively about the importance of client-centred practice and the need for the student to collaborate consistently with the service user who is deemed to be the expert in the occupational therapy process. In order to do this effectively the service user must be viewed holistically, with full consideration to be given to the physical, psychological and social aspects of the individual, see Table 5.9.

Table 5.9 Knowledge about people required for effective intervention
(Adapted from Hocking and Ness, 2002, p. 15)

Knowledge of People
People as occupational beings
Feelings about, reflections on, and interpretations of past, present and future participation in occupation
The relationship between occupation and human development over the lifespan
The relationship between psychological factors and occupation
The relationship between body structures and function and human capacity to participate in occupation
The experience and expression of personal meaning through occupation
How changes or challenges to body structure and function, the course of development, social or cultural disruption, or the personal meaning of occupation may alter people's participation in occupation or their experience of participation
How to manage disruption to body structure or function to preserve the potential to participate in occupation

The student will learn that the intervention skills required for effective intervention related to people are communication, building rapport, negotiation, collaboration, facilitation, etc.

Environment

Finally, the environment is the third aspect that the student must always consider within intervention (see Table 5.10). This can incorporate the physical, social, economic, cultural and political environment that the service user is a part of (Creek, 2003). All play an important part for the student in working with the individual in order to achieve the aims of treatment.

The skills required for effective intervention related to the environment are 'modifying aspects of the human and physical environment to promote participation' (Hocking and Ness, 2002, p.16).

Therefore the complexity of the interplay between the person, the environment and the occupation demonstrate that it is difficult to categorise interventions and present a definitive process that reflects occupational therapy intervention. Students will be expected to apply the theoretical frames of reference and approaches they have learnt in university to provide some foundation of evidence on which to base intervention and so in some part provide this 'category' of interventions.

These are described in more detail below.

Table 5.10 Knowledge and skills related to the environment required for effective intervention. (Adapted from Hocking and Ness, 2002, p. 16)

Knowledge about the Environment
How aspects of the social and cultural environment, such as family, friends, members of the community, employers, teachers, etc. affect people's participation in occupation
How resources in the environment such as the design of buildings, town planning, transport, and playgrounds, and the local geography, etc. affect people's participation in occupation
How aspects of the institutional environment such as institutional racism, apartheid and poverty, affect people's participation in occupation

Frames of Reference and Approaches to Practice

A frame of reference within occupational therapy practice provides the conceptual framework on which practice is based. It has been described by Duncan (2011, p. 45) as 'A theoretical or conceptual idea that has been developed outside the profession but, with judicious use, is applicable within occupational therapy practice'. The approach is then the practical application of this theoretical framework and can provide guidance for the student on applying the theory to practice.

It is crucial for the student to ensure that there is an evidence base for occupational therapy intervention. Although this may not necessarily be overt and transparent within the actual intervention, it is good practice to consider the theoretical framework that is driving the practice.

It is likely that students will discover that occupational therapists use a combination of approaches with one individual, often described as an 'eclectic' approach. The specific approaches are described below with some examples of interventions that may be used within each approach.

Psychological Approaches

Cognitive Behavioural

The cognitive behavioural approach is based on theoretical foundations from the cognitive therapy and behavioural therapy schools of thought. It highlights that our behaviour and thinking are inextricably linked and therefore if behaviour is to be adapted or changed in any way, cognition and patterns of thought have to be addressed.

Ivan Pavlov (1849–1936), John Watson (1878–1958) and Burrhus Skinner (1904–1990) were key theorists in the development of behavioural therapy theoretical foundations, introducing the concepts of classical and operant conditioning. These highlight how behaviour is reinforced both positively and negatively by the consequences to the behaviour.

Interventions that students may learn to use with this approach (see case study 2):

- Anxiety management programmes
- Anger management programmes
- Graded programmes using activities that may trigger stress/anxiety/phobias
- Any activity that incorporates behavioural management techniques, e.g. team working through the activity of canoeing.

Psychodynamic

Sigmund Freud (1856–1939) was the father of the psychodynamic school of thought. His interpretation of human interaction and behaviour was based on the ideology that our subconscious being (our id) drives our conscious behaviour (our ego). He asserted that we are products of our relationships and events in our past, placing great emphasis on our family and parental relationships. In order to resolve this conflict therefore, one must endeavour to strengthen the ego by bringing the unconscious conflicts to the conscious.

The goal of occupational therapy intervention using the psychodynamic approach is therefore to address occupational imbalance caused by subconscious conflict by using therapeutic media to bring the unconscious to the conscious.

Interventions that students may learn to use with this approach (see case study 2):

- Creative therapies, e.g. pottery, art, using 'projective techniques'
- Outdoor activities using reflective techniques
- The use of 'metaphor' that could be applied to many different activities.

Humanistic

Key theorists from the humanistic school of thought include Carl Rogers (1902–1987) and Abraham Maslow (1908–1970). The key concepts that underpin this approach emphasise the importance of empowering the individual through strengthening self-concept and personal growth. Carl Rogers in particular identified that self-esteem is paramount in achieving psychological health, and how we believe others perceive us is a strong determinant of this. Abraham Maslow is most well known for his hierarchy of needs. He asserts that the goal for every individual is to achieve self-actualisation. However, this can only be achieved if each step of the pyramid is achieved in progression, thus identifying the priority given to human needs and motivations.

Interventions that students may learn to use with this approach:

Any intervention may be used with a humanistic perspective, but the skill of the student using this approach will be to empower the individual to achieve 'self actualisation' through setting occupational goals that are truly meaningful. This will clearly be different for each individual but the emphasis will be on the service user's goals, desires, values and motivation. The humanistic approach is the advocate of true client-centred practice.

Tools that may be used in occupational therapy intervention using the humanistic approach:

- Counselling skills – empathy, active listening, reflective questions, etc.
- Positive reinforcement
- Unconditional positive regard.

Physical Approaches

Bio-mechanical

This approach views the body as a functioning machine, made up of specific parts that may be damaged by disease or injury (Foster, 2002). It uses knowledge of activity analysis in order to design treatment regimes to regain function. There is a focus on physical performance. This approach is closely linked to the medical model.

Interventions that students may learn to use with this approach (see case study 3):

- Exercise programmes incorporating functional goals
- Remedial games, e.g. large table top activities to promote/increase range of movement in the upper limb.

Compensatory

The compensatory approach is used widely to compensate for dysfunction and used to enable individuals to pursue their preferred occupations. The compensation may involve adapting the environment, the way an individual performs an activity or provision of equipment/orthoses/information. This is closely linked with the medical model. Duncan (2011) suggests that many occupational therapists favour this approach due to the time restraints and pressure to produce an effective outcome rapidly.

Interventions that students may learn to use with this approach (see case studies 3 and 4):

- Provision of equipment that aids independence, e.g. raised toilet seats, chair raisers, bathboard, etc.
- Adaptation to the physical environment, e.g. walk in shower, ramps, etc.
- Orthoses, e.g. resting splint.

Rehabilitative

The rehabilitative approach considers that a person's ability can be improved through therapeutic intervention. A key element of this approach is that the condition has the potential to be improved. The approach relies heavily on the service user's motivation, not only for independence but also for therapeutic intervention. The rehabilitative approach has been criticised for its requirement for the service user to have a high tolerance and persistence to ensure rehabilitation is effective.

Interventions that students may learn to use with this approach (see case study 4):

- Activities of Daily Living, e.g. washing and dressing
- Remedial activities, e.g. the game of draughts to increase cognitive functioning
- Graded programmes, e.g. increasing or decreasing complexity of requirements from the service user to meet required goal
- Work simulation, e.g. practising specific activities required in the service user's work environment.

Techniques commonly used by the therapist are:

- Cueing: providing a visual or auditory cue to undertake an activity, e.g. verbal prompts, pager, notes, etc. in order to stimulate a response.
- Guiding: physical facilitation, e.g. providing dynamic inhibitory and facilitatory handling during an activity.
- Coaching: psychological facilitation, e.g. developing potential through negotiated goal setting. Also see Chapter 7.

Developmental

This approach has an understanding of human development at the core. It is commonly regarded that development occurs dynamically, so a change in one element impacts upon the other. These elements may be internal: cognition, motor functioning, perception, or external; the environment, socialisation etc.

The approaches of key developmental theorists are all based on these principles but have adopted a specific focus, see Table 5.11.

Table 5.11 Neurological theorists and their focus of approach

Theorist	Focus of Approach
Karel and Bertha Bobath (Raine et al., 2009)	Normal Movement
Jean Ayres (2005)	Sensory Integration
Margaret Rood (1954)	Sensorimotor Integration
Janet Carr and Roberta Sheppard (1998)	Motor Re-learning

Interventions that students may learn to use with this approach:

- Remedial activities
- Activities of daily living, e.g. washing and dressing
- Sensory stimulation, e.g. icing, brushing, vibration, vestibular stimulation
- Sensory integration.

Social Approach

This approach is based on the principle that people are social beings and are influenced by their interaction with the physical and social environment. This is a two-way process and so also recognises the influence that people have on the environment. Social theorists such as Karl Marx (1818–1883), Emile Durkheim (1858–1917) and Max Weber (1864–1920) have been influential in identifying sociology as a discipline in its own right and the complexity of the interaction between society and the individual. Sociological theory is important in informing occupational therapy intervention; if social barriers impact negatively upon participation in occupation, the occupational therapist will use the social approach to address these barriers in order to facilitate occupational engagement. Conversely, social influences can also facilitate occupational performance and the skilled therapist will identify and use these in the intervention programme. The individual is always viewed in the context of their society within this approach.

Interventions that the student may learn to use with this approach:

- Empowering individuals to campaign to reduce stigma of mental health conditions in society.
- Encouraging petitions to local authorities to improve disabled facilities in community buildings.
- Facilitating group interventions to develop social skills.

Four Case Studies Indicating Application of Intervention Approaches on Placement (See Tables 5.12, 5.13, 5.14 and 5.15).

Table 5.12 Case study 1: Child with Duchenne Muscular Dystrophy (DMD)
(With thanks to Jude Pickford)

Background
Simon is 10 years old and lives with his parents and 6-year-old sister on the family farm. He currently attends his local primary school and is going to be moving to secondary school next year. Simon's grandparents live a mile away and provide practical support to him and his family, although his grandmother is becoming increasingly forgetful. Simon is known to the community children's therapy team, which consists of one occupational therapist, one physiotherapist, a speech and language therapist and a therapy support assistant.

Diagnosis and Presentation

Simon was diagnosed with Duchenne Muscular Dystrophy (DMD) when he was 3 years old. His mobility is deteriorating and he has to use a wheelchair intermittently outside although he prefers to be as independently mobile as possible. Simon has very mild learning difficulties but with the help of a support worker he is able to maintain his studies in mainstream education.

Assessment and Planning

From the OT home assessment it was apparent that Simon was finding mobility around the home increasingly difficult and he is finding self-care tasks a struggle. Mobility around school was also difficult, particularly in the school playground; Simon was becoming more fatigued in the afternoon. Simon is very sociable and enjoys spending time with his friends.

Long term aim (identified by Simon):

>   To do as much as I can on my own, on the farm and with my friends.

Short term aims: To help out more on the farm

>   To go to Dave's swimming party

>   To feel safer in the playground at break

>   To get ready for school myself

>   To be able to write more easily.

Choice of Interventions and Justification

Short term aim	Intervention	Justification	Approach Used
To help out more on the farm	Design posters for new vegetable box venture	Small adapted equipment (built up pen and writing board) and use of assistive technology can be introduced for a meaningful occupation.	Compensatory
To go to Dave's swimming party	Graded approach of one-to-one swimming sessions (with rehab assistant), then a swimming session with his mum and friends in order to work towards swimming party.	Joint working with physiotherapist to establish optimum exercise level. As well as encouraging Simon to reach developmental milestones, this activity will provide physical exercise, and begin to address any barriers to community participation.	Social Developmental

To feel safer in the playground at breaktime.	The student will identify a playground game (e.g. hide and seek) that will be suitable for Simon's physical ability and encourage social interaction. This will be graded with a small group of peers initially.	Developmentally Simon should be engaging in peer and competitive team play (Case Smith 2001). A graded approach will encourage development of confidence and use his strength of high social functioning (Kohler et al., 2005). Use this as a vehicle to educate Simon's peers and teachers if necessary.	Adaptive Developmental Educational Social
To get ready for school myself	The student will initially explore non-equipment based adaptive techniques. Gradually educate re: equipment and fatigue management strategies and introduce discreet measures: e.g. use of perching stool in bathroom	Although Simon does not want to use equipment, it is important to explore why and address fears around this.	Compensatory Educational
To be able to write more easily	The student will introduce Simon to adapted tools – e.g. built up pen and writing board. Educate re: importance of posture – e.g. optimum pelvic position (Kramer and Hinojosa, 2009)	Joint working with the support worker to introduce these strategies will help to develop Simon's confidence in handwriting and reduce fatigue.	Educational Compensatory Developmental

Table 5.13 Case study 2: Female adolescent with anorexia nervosa
(With thanks to Daune Gregorian)
NB. As this case study is in a specialist area the student may need closer supervision direction than in other settings.

Background
Jessica is 16, and lives at home with her mother and stepfather. Her father (who she had a good relationship with) left home when she was 7 and she has not seen him since. She has a very volatile relationship with both her mother and stepfather and insists that they do not understand how she feels. She spends a lot of time on her own in her room, listening to music. She has very few friends at school and tends to be very socially withdrawn.

Diagnosis and Presentation
Jessica has recently been diagnosed with anorexia nervosa. She is 5'6" tall and weighs 6 stone. She does not eat breakfast or lunch and eats a minimal amount of dinner under her parents' supervision who now monitor her food intake. She insists on walking everywhere to get as much exercise as she can. She is irritable and withdrawn and often experiences panic attacks when in social situations, particularly if there is food involved.

Choice of Intervention and Justification
Jessica has been referred to an occupational therapy programme within the CAMHs service to address her eating disorder. Following an initial assessment by the student, supervised by the occupational therapist, the key strengths and needs are identified and a programme of activities is negotiated in collaboration with Jessica. The therapeutic relationship is paramount at this stage as Jessica is not at the unit out of her own choice. Clear and effective communication by the student is therefore key in developing a rapport that is based on trust and empathy and able to draw on the complex nature of Jessica's goals. Following a period of negotiation the following programme of activities is agreed upon and a contract signed. Within this contract there are a number of 'non-negotiables' that Jessica must sign up to (Geller and Srikameswaran, 2006).

Day and Time	Activity	Description	Approach Used
Monday am	Food preparation Meal planning	Initially Jessica is encouraged by the student to observe and smell/touch the food to allow exposure and reduce anxiety in being around food. Jessica is encouraged to discuss her fear of food within this activity. Focus is on the sensory experience of food preparation.	Cognitive behavioural Sensory integration

Monday pm	Relaxation	Jessica participates in a relaxation session led by the student where she learns positive coping techniques to manage her anxiety and relax.	Educational
Wednesday am	Food preparation Meal planning	Jessica is encouraged by the student to cook a healthy and nutritious meal advised by her dietician. She will then eat this with her group at lunchtime. The student will continue to sensitively encourage Jessica to name her anxieties and fears through this process.	Cognitive Behavioural
Wednesday pm	Creative activities	Jessica is encouraged to participate in a therapeutic creative activity led by the student where 'projection techniques' are adopted to identify triggers to low self esteem. Activities include art, pottery, collages ,etc.	Psychodynamic
Friday am	Food preparation Meal planning Budgeting	Jessica is given a budget and the student supports her along with her group to purchase a meal and cook her own lunch independently. She is encouraged to cook a nutritious well-balanced meal, following the advice of her dietician. Anxieties continue to be addressed and gently challenged in this process.	Cognitive Behavioural
Friday pm	Community activity	Jessica and her group are encouraged to undertake activities in the community to encourage 'normalisation' of body image – e.g. shopping for clothes, whilst identifying good coping strategies and challenging irrational and negative thoughts. Jessica is also encouraged to practice eating out in the community, and this activity is graded – e.g. eating sandwiches as a picnic to eating in a cafe. These skills can be transferred back to her school environment.	Cognitive Behavioural

Monthly	Family therapy session	Family are offered a joint therapy session to explore family dynamics and reinforce the work that is done at the unit (Treasure *et al.* 2007).	Psycho-educational

At the start of each day Jessica is given a goal setting sheet by the student where she is encouraged to set small achievable goals for the day. These are reviewed at the end of the day. All activities are undertaken in a relaxed manner in groups up to eight people. Initially Jessica struggled with this due to her fear of social situations but with reassurance that this was a 'safe place' and as she started to make a couple of good friends within the unit her confidence grows. During the three days that she is at the unit Jessica is encouraged to eat her breakfast and lunch with the rest of the group. This is approached sensitively and staff aim to provide emotional support throughout the process. The programme is graded and flexible to ensure a client-centred approach is adopted and is therefore effective and transferable to Jessica's home situation.

Table 5.14 Case study 3: Female adult with osteoarthritis in carpometacarpal joint.
(With thanks to Ruth Squire)

Background and Diagnosis
Audrey is a 45-year-old podiatrist who lives with her husband and two children. She is fit and healthy apart from experiencing a painful right thumb. She has been referred to the hand unit for splinting by her GP, who has diagnosed osteoarthritis.

Current Presentation
On assessment, Audrey reports that she manages most occupations herself apart from some tasks in the kitchen, which cause her pain at the base of her right thumb in the carpometacarpal joint (CMC). She reports that her main concern is how the condition is limiting her work, as some days she is unable to use her tools to treat her patients. Audrey is keen to continue working.

Intervention and Justification
The Hand Therapy Unit that Audrey is referred to consists of a small team of specialist occupational and physiotherapists, and is attached to the trauma and orthopaedic outpatient department. Initially, the student observes the occupational therapist carried out a variety of hand assessments to establish baseline levels in Audrey's function, pain, strength and range of movement. Interventions carried out by the occupational therapist with Audrey included splinting, advice regarding functional limitation, how to increase independence, strengthening work. Audrey was seen for a number of sessions over four weeks.

Intervention and Approach
In order that Audrey is able to maintain and improve her ability both at work and whilst carrying out tasks in the kitchen, the student with the support of the OT will use a blend of underpinning approaches including biomechanical and compensatory principles.
Biomechanically, the student teaches Audrey strengthening exercises using therapeutic putty, which will help to provide support and improve the range of movement for the affected area. Care must be taken to teach Audrey how to monitor her pain threshold as too much exercise may increase her pain levels. The student encourages Audrey to make use of her meaningful occupations to increase her grip strength, for example baking. Support for the painful joint can be given in the form of a thermoplastic splint, which the student and the OT will either customise for Audrey or provide her with an off the shelf version. The splint is worn while she carries out specific duties/tasks which cause pain, enabling Audrey to carry on with the task in more comfort.
In order that Audrey can carry on using the tools of her trade, the student and OT provide her with some adaptations, like building up the handles on the nail cutting tool with insulation tubing to reduce the pressure on the base of the thumb. Here the student follows compensatory principles, as they are adapting the environment in order that Audrey can be independent. Other adaptive equipment ideas are shown to Audrey in relation to the difficulties experienced in the kitchen. These include use of an electric tin opener, a 'jar key', and lever style taps to help reduce pain in her CMC joint.
Intervention will be complete when Audrey reports that she can manage her work and kitchen tasks with less pain and that she has learnt how to manage her condition.

Table 5.15 Case study 4: Male older adult with total hip replacement after a fall

Background and Diagnosis
Mr Jones is 78 years old. He lives alone in a two storey privately owned house on the edge of a village. The bedroom and bathroom are upstairs, but there is a toilet downstairs. He was discharged from hospital this morning following a two week hospital admission after falling and fracturing his right neck of femur. He had a total hip replacement and has made a good recovery. Prior to hospital admission Mr Jones was fully independent and did not receive any services.
He has been referred to the re-ablement team for six weeks with the aim to increase his overall level of independence. The re-ablement occupational therapist and student visited Mr Jones in hospital and have liaised closely with the hospital occupational therapists to ensure a smooth transition of care.

Current Presentation
Walks (indoors only) with the aid of a zimmer frame. Trendelenburg gait. Transfers from a high chair, bed and toilet (with Mowbray frame) with difficulty. Unable to safely climb the stairs. Requires some assistance with personal care; particularly the lower half. Able to make a hot drink and simple snack if all equipment within easy reach. No cognitive impairment. Very motivated.

Intervention and Justification
A six week re-ablement service to consist of 10 sessions per week (Monday–Friday). Family have agreed to offer support on the weekends. This intensive programme can be used to offer a graded programme and the nature of the service means that Mr Jones will be supported in increasing his independence in all his occupational domains.

Intervention and Approach
The programme will incorporate rehabilitation and compensatory approaches to address the issues highlighted in 'Current Presentation' above. The programme will initially start with an early morning visit to work with Mr Jones to improve his independence with getting up from bed, washing and dressing. This will incorporate a graded programme (rehabilitation approach) increasing in complexity.
Initially Mr Jones will use the dressing aids provided and the zimmer frame to assist with mobility (compensation approach). Mr Jones will be taught techniques for safe transfers and dressing. Mr Jones will then make himself a simple breakfast and have a rest period. At lunchtime the student will return to assist Mr Jones in preparing a hot meal. Again this will be graded in complexity and time required. The physiotherapist will also provide a home programme of exercises to increase Mr Jones's strength, mobility and range of movement (biomechanical). These will be practised regularly throughout the day. As Mr Jones's independence improves the equipment will be removed when it is no longer needed. Once Mr Jones has increased his mobility to walking with a stick the student can progress the programme to Mr Jones resuming activities outside of the house, e.g. shopping, leisure, etc. Initially this will start with escorted activities, progressing to independence (rehabilitation).

Conclusion

This section of the chapter has aimed to introduce some of the principles of occupational therapy intervention along with a selection of frames of references and theoretical approaches that the student occupational therapist is likely to encounter during practice placements. Four case studies have applied some of these principles and theories to illustrate their use in occupational therapy intervention.

Reflective Questions

1. What range of interventions have you experienced on your practice placements so far?

- How occupationally focused were they?
- How client-centred were they?
- How did the environment play a part in the intervention?

2. Consider what approaches you have used within your interventions on placement so far.

- What did these look like in practice?
- How effective were they?

3. How might you transfer your intervention skills from one placement to another?

References

Ayres, A.J. (2005) *Sensory Integration and the Child: 25th Anniversary Edition*. Los Angeles: Cresport Press.

Carr, J.H. and Shepherd, R. (1998) *Neurological Rehabilitation: Optimizing Motor Performance*. Oxford: Butterworth-Heinemann.

Case-Smith, J. (2001) 'Development of Childhood Occupations' in J. Case-Smith (ed.) *Occupational Therapy for Children*. London: Mosby, pp. 71–94.

Creek, J. (2003) *Occupational Therapy Defined as a Complex Intervention*. London: College of Occupational Therapists.

Duncan, E.A.S. (2011) 'An introduction to models and conceptual frameworks of practice' in E.A.S. Duncan (ed.) *Foundations for Practice in Occupational Therapy* (5th Edition) Edinburgh: Elsevier, pp. 43–48.

Foster, M. (2002) 'Theoretical Frameworks'. In A. Turner, M. Foster, and S.E. Johnson (eds) *Occupational Therapy and Physical Dysfunction* (5th Edition). London: Churchill Livingstone, pp.47–84.

Geller, J., and Srikameswaran, S, (2006) 'Treatment non negotiables: Why we need them and how to make them work'. *European Eating Disorders Review*, **14** (4) 212–217.

Hocking, C., and Ness, N.E. (2002) *Revised Minimum Standards for the Education of Occupational Therapists*. Australia: World Federation of Occupational Therapists.

Kohler, M., Clarenbach, C.F., Boni, L., Brack, T., Russi, E.R., and Bloch, K.E. (2005) 'Quality of life, physical disability, and respiratory impairment in Duchenne Muscular Dystrophy'. *American Journal of Respiratory Critical Care Medicine*, **172**: 1032–1036.

Kramer, P., and Hinojosa, J. (2009) *Frames of Reference for Pediatric Occupational Therapy* (3rd ed.) London: Wolters Kluwer, Lippincott Williams & Wilkins.

Raine, S., Meadows, L. and Lynch-Ellerington, M. (2009) *Bobath Concept: Theory and Clinical Practice in Neurological Rehabilitation*. London: Wiley Blackwell.

Rood, M.S. (1954) 'Neurophysiology reactions as a basis for physical therapy'. *Physical Therapy Review*, **34**: 444–449.

Sumsion, T. (2006) *Client-Centred Practice in Occupational Therapy: A guide to implementation*. Second Edition. London: Churchill Livingstone.

Treasure, J., Smith, G.D., and Crane, A.M. (2007) *Skills Based Learning for Caring for a Loved One with an Eating Disorder: The New Maudsley Method*. London: Routledge.

Watson, R. and Swartz, L. (2004) *Transformation through Occupation*. London: Whurr Publishers Ltd.

Section 4:
Evaluation Knowledge and Skills on Placement
Rachel Treseder and Tracey Polglase

Introduction

It is important that students learn the skills of evaluation through their practice education. There are many different methods of evaluating practice and this section will cover the principles of evaluation and different tools that may be used to evaluate practice. Four case studies will be used with specific examples of evaluation techniques, e.g. standardised and non-standardised evaluation tools.

Principles of Evaluation

Creek (2010, p. 25) defines evaluation as 'The process of obtaining, interpreting and appraising information (about occupational performance) in order to prioritise problems and needs, to plan and modify interventions and to judge the worth of interventions.'

Evaluation is the final stage of the occupational therapy process, although it may also be an integral part of the process at each stage after assessment as indicated in Creek's definition above. It is a crucial element of occupational therapy practice to ensure that the goals set at the assessment and planning stage have been met and practice is reviewed accordingly.

Why evaluate?
- To measure progress or deterioration
- To provide evidence
- To ensure quality
- To assist in decision making
- To plan effectively.

As with assessment, evaluation can be standardised or non-standardised and so a number of formal and informal tools can be used. This section of the chapter will aim to discuss some of these.

Evaluating the Service User
Non-standardised evaluation tools

Just as information was gathered at initial referral from a variety of sources, it is important that this is maintained throughout the problem solving process. In order to inform the evaluation of the outcome the student can gather information from the following sources:

Patient's medical notes

Information that has been recorded in the medical notes will present a valuable picture of the progress of the service user since initial contact. This will contribute to the overall evaluation of the service user and must be used to fully evaluate the progress using a holistic inter-professional approach.

Relatives/friends

Relatives and friends can continue to provide valuable information at the evaluation stage of the process. Their perspective may provide alternative/additional information to what the student/ professional has observed. However, as with the assessment stage, consent must be gained from the service user prior to contacting the family/friends unless their capacity to consent has been assessed and they are deemed not to have capacity.

Other professionals

The multi-disciplinary team will provide valuable information on the progress of the service user since the assessment stage. Again the student will gain a more holistic picture of the service user at the point of evaluation. There may be professionals from other services and organisations that may contribute to the evaluation process although the service user must be informed that evaluation outcomes will be shared with the wider team and professionals.

Observation

Just as important information could be gathered from observation at the assessment stage, the same is true at the evaluation stage. There is a wealth of information that can be gained from observing a service user repeat an activity that they completed at the assessment stage. Although not a standardised evaluation tool, the student can use his/her skills of observation to record the progress of the service user, and thus evidence the impact of occupational therapy intervention.

Service user verbal feedback

The therapeutic alliance between the student and the service user is instrumental to the whole process and this has been consistently highlighted in the previous chapters. This remains true at the evaluation stage and one of the most important methods of evaluating effectiveness is to gather verbal feedback from the service user. It is important that the service user has the opportunity to comment on the quality of occupational therapy intervention, how effective they feel this intervention has been, and their interpretation of the outcomes. This verbal feedback may often present a different picture to the student's perceived outcome, and so it is imperative that the service user is given the opportunity to express his/her views.

Questionnaires

Service users can also be given an opportunity to express their opinions in a written manner using questionnaires. These can come in a variety of forms:

Satisfaction surveys

These tend to be multiple-choice questionnaires using closed questions that aim to quantify the service user's opinions on particular aspects of the service given. Satisfaction surveys are usually used for a wider population and the statistics used to modify and improve services. Service users should be assured of anonymity and confidentiality so that they feel free to express their opinions openly.

Evaluation questionnaires

This form of questionnaire is usually more qualitative in nature and so aims to gather more in-depth information about the experience of the service user. Although they may not necessarily be anonymous, the service user is given much more opportunity to express their experience rather than merely ticking a box. This may also serve as a reflective tool for the service user to gain insight into progress made.

Standardised Evaluation Tools

Assessment tools

Any of the standardised assessment tools discussed earlier in this chapter may be repeated by the student after occupational therapy intervention to review progress of the service user. There are specific criteria for the timescale for some of these and this should always be followed in order for the results to be valid.

Outcome Measures

Students may have the opportunity to use outcome measures during their placement. Outcome measures are standardised tools that aim to 'quantify the change in a patient or population as a result of preceding intervention.' (Clarke *et al.*, 2001 p. 3). As the name suggests their main purpose is to measure the outcome of intervention in a quantifiable manner. They serve to improve care by using evidence-based practice and ensuring client-centred practice. The College of Occupational Therapists have developed a comprehensive guide to the use of outcome measures (Clarke *et al.*, 2001) but the following table aims to give an overview of some of the measures that students may find are used in practice today.

OT specific and generic outcome measures

The following table (5.16) summarise, some of the specific outcome measures that are used in occupational therapy practice, followed by some more generic outcome measures that are utilised (Table 5.17).

Table 5.16 OT specific outcome measures

Name of Standardised Outcome Measure	Clinical Area/ Life Cycle Stage	Additional Information
Assessment of Motor Process Skills (AMPS) (Fisher, 1995)	All areas	Observational assessment of occupational performance. Specific training required
AusTOMS (Unsworth and Duncombe, 2004)	All areas	Service user function is rated in four areas: Impairment, Activity Limitation, Participation Restriction and Distress/ Well-being Guidelines are provided but additional training not required
Canadian Occupational Performance Measure (Law et al., 2005)	All areas	Emphasis is on client-centred practice with opportunity for collaborative goal setting. Accompanied with training manual – training is recommended although not essential
Chessington Occupational Therapy Neurological Assessment Battery (COTNAB) (Tyerman et al., 1986)	Neurology	Designed to assess and evaluate functional ability of neurology service users – i.e. visual perception, constructional ability, sensorimotor ability
Morriston Occupational Therapy Outcome Measure (James and Corr, 2004)	Any area where the focus is on occupational performance	Five point rating scale that measures occupational performance. Training not required but a comprehensive user manual has been developed
Rivermead Activities of Daily Living (Whiting and Lincoln, 1980)	Neurology (stroke)	Evaluates the recovery of activity of daily living (ADL) skills for service users following a stroke or head injury
Volitional Questionnaire (VQ) (De las Heras et al., 2007)	Any area	Used in conjunction with Model of Human Occupation (Kielhofner, 2008) and is designed to assess level of motivation in specific areas

Model of Human Occupation Screening Tool Version 2.0 (MOHOST) (Parkinson et al., 2006)	A variety of settings	Used to screen for occupational therapy services and document progress from intervention – covers the key concepts from the Model of Human Occupation (Kielhofner, 2008)
Occupational Self Assessment (OSA) (Baron et al., 2006)	A variety of settings	A self-assessment tool that records a service user's perceived ability and motivation for identified occupations
Functional Independence Measure Functional Assessment Measure (FIM/FAM) (Dittmar and Granger, 1997)	Neurology and brain injury	Service users are rated on their need for assistance

Table 5.17 Generic outcome measures

Name of Standardised Outcome Measure	Clinical Area/Life Cycle Stage	Additional Information
Barthel Self Care Index (Shah et al., 1989)	Physical disability Elderly care Neurology Rheumatology	Measure of functional independence in personal care and mobility
Becks Depression Inventory (BDI-II) (Beck et al., 1996)	Mental Health Paediatrics	Clinical assessment and screening of depression
Clifton Assessment Procedures for the Elderly (CAPE) (Pattie and Gilleard, 1979)	Elderly Mental Health	Consists of two parts – Cognitive Assessment Scale and Behaviour Rating Scale
Hospital Anxiety and Depression scale (Snaith and Zigmond, 1994)	All areas	Self report measure – designed to distinguish effects of physical illness from mild mood disorder

Mayer's Lifestyle Questionnaire (Mayers, 1993)	Community, particularly social services	Designed to reflect a broad assessment of need and quality of life as perceived by the service user
Middlesex Elderly Assessment of Mental State (MEAMS) (Golding, 1989)	Elderly Mental Health Physical Neurology	Designed to distinguish between organic and functional illnesses particularly with the elderly
Mini Mental State Examination (MMSE) (Folstein et al., 1975)	Elderly Neurology Mental Health	A measure of cognitive performance – frequently used to assist in diagnosing dementia. Easy and quick to administer

Evaluating the Service

Evaluation also involves measuring the service provision as a whole in addition to the progress of the service user. The aims are still to ensure quality of care and evidence-based practice. There are a number of tools that can be used in evaluating the service.

Research

Students are entering an arena where occupational therapists are required to work within an evidence-based practice culture. Empirical and literature based research provides the evidence that informs practice. The COT code of ethics and professional conduct (2010) requires occupational therapists to be research active and base their professional practice on sound evidence that has been rigorously evaluated and researched. The student may have a significant role during placement in providing evidence of current research from their studies.

Audit

Audit is a process of monitoring performance using specific criteria to measure against. The student may be aware of specific audits that are being carried out on services during their placement. There are a range of tools that can be used for this purpose in order to meet the specific needs. Audit is often a cyclical process whereby specific performance is measured, reviewed, modified and measured again. Below is a list of tools that can be used under the audit umbrella:

- Peer Review: auditing of performance by a peer/colleague using a set criterion in order to further develop skills and expertise.
- Organisational Audit: evaluation by conducting a survey of standards concerned with systems and processes for the delivery of healthcare.
- Criterion Audit: Measuring achievements against standards. Audit of the service.
- Standards Review: e.g. Health Professions Council audit of continuing professional development.
- Meeting target levels set in contracts: this may be monitored at the annual service review with the key stakeholders.

Benchmarking

Benchmarking is a process that uses a number of organisations in a collaborative arrangement in order to improve quality of service. The organisations involved measure their own performance against each other to seek out best practice. Specific targets are stipulated in relation to performance, efficiency and effectiveness. The College of Occupational Therapists have a number of publications that incorporate benchmarking procedures for specialist areas of practice and professional development (see http://www.cot.co.uk/find/node/benchmarking).

Case Studies Indicating Use of Evaluation on Placement

(See Tables 5.18, 5.19, 5.20 and 5.21)

Table 5.18 Case study 1: Forensic adult mental health (with thanks to Nicole Burchett)

Background and presenting features
Michael is a 22-year-old male in a medium secure unit. He was admitted to the unit where, following conviction he was detained for attempted murder during a psychotic episode. He also has a history of drug and alcohol abuse. He has no contact with his family and has a 2-year-old son, whom he has not seen for 6 months since the breakdown in relationship with the mother. He does not appear to have established any friendships since being at the secure unit.
Assessment and intervention
Following establishing a rapport with Michael, the student completed an initial assessment using the (OPHI) to obtain his history. During this assessment Michael appears low in mood and agitated. The student then used the Occupational Self Assessment (OSA) tool (Baron et al., 2006) with Michael. This indicated that he had little motivation for most occupations, and had difficulties in establishing friendships and communicating effectively with people. He was, however, interested in gardening as his grandfather had taken him to his allotment as a child before he died suddenly 10 years ago.

Following a number of risk assessments completed by the multi-disciplinary team, including the HCR-20 (Webster et al., 1997) and mental health relapse indicators, the student (with assistance from the occupational therapist) completed a number of one to one sessions with Michael in the unit's garden plot. As he receives input from other members of the MDT (psychiatrist, psychologist, nurse) and his mood elevates, Michael agrees to attend the gardening group with five other members. Within this group he is given opportunity to express anger positively, establish friendships over a shared activity, and develop productivity by working towards a specific goal.

Evaluation Tools and Justification

Twelve weeks after the initial assessment the student repeated the OSA with Michael. This information was used to write a report for the multidisciplinary peer review at this stage.

The OSA indicated that there were a number of factors that he was beginning to recognise the need to work on, namely taking care of himself, getting along with others, relaxing and enjoying himself, and doing activities that he liked. In addition there were other factors that, although he did not feel he had improved in, he recognised had become more important to him. These included managing his finances, expressing himself to others, handling responsibility and using his abilities effectively. This assessment tool used as an outcome measure demonstrated Michael's increased insight and potential for development in motivation for specific tasks which provided opportunity for the student to work in collaboration with Michael to set new goals for future intervention. The OSA would be used to review Michael's progress again in 6 months.

Table 5.19 Case study 2: Psychiatry of old age

Background and presenting features

Elsie is 78 years old and lives with her older sister Lily, 85, for whom she is the primary carer. Her only son and his wife live 150 miles away and try to visit every two months. Her niece visits once a week to take her shopping. Over the last six months Elsie has become increasingly forgetful, and repeats herself in conversation. She has limited insight into this. She has also been forgetting to do important tasks at home and has missed important appointments. Her sister has expressed concern to the niece and son and so after an initial appointment with the GP she has been referred to the Community Mental Health team.

Assessment and intervention

On initial assessment the student gathered information from Elsie's medical history and with permission spoke to her sister, niece and son. Communication with the multi-disciplinary team at the assessment stage also enabled a holistic approach.

Elsie was diagnosed with early stage dementia and the student (with support from the occupational therapist) was asked to carry out a Middlesex Elderly Assessment Measure (MEAMS) to determine the nature and severity of cognitive impairment (Golding, 1989). This indicated that Elsie was scoring within the borderline range meaning that her cognitive impairment required monitoring more closely, and further assessment was important.

A functional kitchen assessment also indicated that Elsie was still able to function well and safely in the kitchen, although it was acknowledged there may have been an element of risk in relation to using the gas cooker, particularly at certain times of the day.

Elsie was prescribed Aricept medication by the consultant psychiatrist and referred to the memory group run by the community psychiatric nurse (CPN) and occupational therapist in partnership with the Alzheimer's Society. Her niece supported her in attending and transferring new knowledge and information to the home environment. Her goals of intervention were to minimise risk at home and use memory aids and prompts to remain living safely and independently at home for as long as possible.

Evaluation tools and justification

Approximately one month after the eight-week memory group the student evaluated Elsie's progress at home. She gathered information from the family using an evaluation questionnaire that the occupational therapist had developed to determine their perspective on the outcome of the intervention programme. This helped to create a more holistic picture of Elsie's functional ability and safety within the home. The student also repeated the functional assessment in the kitchen to determine whether Elsie had transferred any of the new information from the memory group to her living environment. The MEAMs was repeated to determine whether there had been any further cognitive decline since the original assessment four months earlier.

All of these evaluation tools, both standardised and non-standardised, helped to indicate that intervention had been effective to some extent as Elsie was adopting some of the techniques within the home to aid her memory. This was indicated by the observation of her completing a task and confirmed by the family. The MEAMS suggested that there had been limited cognitive decline since the initial assessment. This information was communicated back to the MDT and confirmed by input from the CPN.

Table 5.20 Case study 3: Palliative care (with thanks to Alison Docherty)

Background and presenting features

Annette is 47 years of age. She lives with her husband and her two children who are 11 and 15 years old. She is currently employed as a teacher in a primary school. She has no extended family living nearby.

She lives in a three storey, detached property and the access is level via a driveway. The ground floor is open plan, there are three bedrooms and a bathroom on the first floor and the master bedroom with an en suite bathroom is on the top floor.

Annette was diagnosed with right sided breast cancer two years ago and had a mastectomy with lymph node removal, followed by radiotherapy and chemotherapy. She developed Lymphoedema in her right arm. She is now presenting with bone metastases within the spine and lung metastases. She has reduced mobility due to pain on movement and increased breathlessness. This has led to reduced abilities to carry out activities of daily living.

Assessment and intervention

Occupational therapy assessments undertaken were daily living assessments including social and psychological components, and mobility and transfer assessments within the specialist hospital palliative care service. The student also undertook a home visit with Annette to assess her within her home environment.

Goals identified

1. To be able to transfer on/off toilet independently.

2. To be able to transfer on/off lounge chair independently.

3. To be able to transfer from supine to sit in bed independently.

4. To be able to manage breathlessness and reduce anxiety.

5. To be able to manage disease related fatigue.

6. To be able to manage personal care with minimal assistance.

7. To be able to manage feeding independently.

8. To be able to manage limited range of domestic activities.

9. To be able to address end of life issues with children.

Intervention

1. The student and the OT provided equipment to enable Annette to transfer on/off toilet independently. Consideration needed to be made as Annette has reduced movement and function in her right arm due to the Lymphoedema. A floor fixed toilet frame and raised toilet seat were fitted.

2. Annette was unable to transfer from her lounge sofa due to the height of the sofa and her reduced function in her arm and her back pain. The student was unable to raise the sofa due to the design and therefore an electric riser recliner chair was provided.

cont.

3. Annette was sleeping in a large queen size bed that consisted of two single beds joined together with two independent single mattresses. It was extremely important to Annette to continue sleeping with her husband. The bed was brought down on to the first floor of the property to enable Annette to access her bedroom via one flight of stairs rather than two. An electric mattress elevator was fitted to Annette's half of the bed.

4. Annette was provided with techniques to self manage some of her breathing difficulties. Anxiety management techniques were also used to help reduce her anxiety levels and a relaxation technique was taught and a CD was issued.

5. Information regarding energy conservation, pacing and fatigue was discussed with both Annette and her husband.

6. Equipment was provided for the shower and home care was organised to support Annette with personal ADL.

7. Large handled cutlery was provided to enable Annette to feed herself independently.

8. A perch stool and adaptive kitchen equipment was provided to enable participation in some domestic activities.

9. The OT and student discussed end of life issues with Annette and facilitated the creation of memory boxes for each of the children.

Evaluation tools and justification

Within this palliative care setting AUSTOMS (Unsworth and Duncombe, 2004) was used as the outcome/evaluation tool, and following OT intervention the scoring demonstrated a significant improvement in the activity participation, and her distress levels were also considerably reduced, even though the service user's physical abilities did not improve overall. The goals set were also reviewed in order to measure effectiveness of intervention.

Evaluation of occupational therapy intervention within the palliative care speciality can present challenges. These challenges are directly related to the outcome/evaluation tool used. Many of the standardised tools available for measuring outcomes of intervention are based on physical function. Palliative care service users by the nature of their diagnosis may have limited opportunity for physical improvement and even when there is physical improvement this may be short lived and will ultimately deteriorate. This deterioration would be highlighted on functional based measures and could demonstrate a negative outcome. Therefore outcome measures/evaluation tools should be sensitive to the holistic nature of palliative care intervention. The outcome measure should incorporate activity or task participation rating and also a scale regarding psychological well-being of the service user.

Table 5.21 Case study 4: Social services

Background and presenting features
John is 36 years old and lives with his wife and three children; who are 5, 8 and 11. They live in a three bedroom semi-detached property with bathroom and toilet upstairs. John was diagnosed with multiple sclerosis 10 years ago. He has deteriorated in the last two years is now struggling to get up the stairs and to use the bathroom facilities. His mobility is poor and he has had a number of falls. He is ataxic and has an intention tremor. He has been referred to the social services occupational therapist for an assessment.

Assessment and intervention
When the occupational therapist and student visited they undertook a thorough environmental assessment and a functional assessment. In light of John's diagnosis it was felt that interventions for the present needed to be considered and proceedings for the future needed to be started, as he was likely to deteriorate further. The student's aim was to improve John's safety and independence in the short term and the long term. Following the assessment the OT and student completed a Disabled Facilities Grant (DFG) application for a ground floor extension to provide a wet room with toileting facilities and a bedroom. In addition a stair-lift was requested to access the first floor prior to this work taking place. The DFG works were on a priority grant and so required a case conference and were allocated to a grants officer within six weeks. The works were then likely to take a further 12 weeks to complete so interim measures also needed to be taken. Advice was also given on how to reduce hazards within the home, e.g. removing of clutter, clearing walkways, removing rugs etc.

Evaluation tools and justification
A range of evaluation tools and procedures were used. **Monitoring**: The OT and student monitored the DFG process throughout by liaising with the DFG department to ensure the grant was processing prior to the start of the build. Once the build started the OT and student visited the site to ensure the plans were progressing as expected. During this time they also liaised with John and his family to address issues and ensure they were happy. **Client Satisfaction Survey**: At the end of the process John was given a client satisfaction survey to complete. This was an opportunity for him and his family to comment upon the DFG process and the quality of service from the OTs.

cont.

105

> **Measurement against Aim**: One month after the hazards were removed and the stair lift installed the OT reviewed John. He reported in the last month he had experienced no further falls and was independently and safely ascending and descending the stairs.
>
> Once the works were completed the OT assessed John using the new ground floor facilities. It was evident that the increase in independence and safety that this offered him also had a consequential impact on the carer role of his wife. She needed to do a lot less for him and was less worried about him injuring himself.

Conclusion

This section of the chapter has aimed to present some of the principles of evaluation within occupational therapy practice that are important for the student to learn throughout their placement experience. It has discussed methods of evaluation for both the service delivery, the professional development of the student and the outcome of intervention with the service user. Four case studies have been used to illustrate the use of some of these evaluation tools in practice.

Reflective Questions

1. What range of evaluation tools have you observed/used on placement?
2. How effective were they in identifying the outcome of occupational therapy intervention?
3. What skills did you need to use the evaluation tool? What further specific experience do you feel you need?
4. How might you transfer skills of evaluation to future placements/practice?

References

Baron, K., Kielhofner, G., Lyenger, A., Goldhammer, V., and Wolenski, J., (2006) *Occupational Self Assessment Version 2.2.* Available at http://www.uic.edu/depts/moho/assess/osa.html (accessed 26/04/12).

Beck, A.T., Steer, R.A., Ball, R., and Ranieri, W. (1996) 'Comparison of Beck Depression Inventories -IA and -II in psychiatric outpatients'. *Journal of Personality Assessment*, **67** (3): 588–97.

Clarke, C., Sealey-Lapes, C., and Kotsch, L. (2001) *Outcome Measures Information Pack for Occupational Therapy.* London: College of Occupational Therapists.

College of Occupational Therapists (2010) *Code of Ethics and Professional Conduct.* London: College of Occupational Therapists.

College of Occupational Therapists (2012) *Benchmarking.* available at http://www.cot.co.uk/find/node/benchmarking (accessed 26/4/12).

Creek, J. (2010) *The Core Concepts of Occupational Therapy: A Dynamic Framework for Practice*. London: Jessica Kingsley Publishers.

De las Heras, C.G., Geist, R., Kielhofner, G., and Li, Y. (2007) *Volitional Questionnaire*. 4th edition. Available at http://www.uic.edu/depts/moho/assess/vq.html (accessed 26/04/12).

Dittmar, S.S., and Granger, G.E. (1997) *Functional Assessment and Outcome Measures for the Rehabilitation Health Professional*. Maryland: Aspen, pp. 7–9.

Fisher, A.G. (1995). *Assessment of Motor and Process Skills* (3rd ed). Fort Collins, CO: Three Star Press.

Folstein, M.F., Folstein, S.E., and McHugh, P.R. (1975) 'Mini-mental state: A practical method for grading the cognitive state of patients for the clinician'. *Journal of Psychiatric Research*, **12**: 189–198.

Golding, E. (1989) *Middlesex Elderly Assessment of Mental State (MEAMS)*. Essex: Pearson Education Ltd.

James, S., and Corr, S. (2004) 'The Morriston Occupational Therapy Outcome Measure (MOTOM): Measuring what matters'. *British Journal of Occupational Therapy*, **67**(5): 210–216.

Kielhofner, G. (2008). *Model of Human Occupation: Theory and Application* (4th edn). Philadelphia: Lippincott, Williams & Wilkins.

Law, M., Baptiste, S., Carswell, A., McColl, M., Polatajko, H., and Pollock, N. (2005) *Canadian Occupational Performance Measure* (4th ed). Ottawa: Canadian Association of Occupational Therapists.

Mayer, C. (1993) 'A model for community occupational therapy practice, stage 1'. *British Journal of Occupational Therapy*, **56**(5): 169–172.

Parkinson, S., Forsyth, K., and Kielhofner, G. (2006) *Model of Human Occupation Screening Tool: Version 2.0*. Available at http://www.uic.edu/depts/moho/assess/mohost.html (accessed 26/04/12).

Pattie, A., and Gilleard, C. (1979) *Clifton Assessment Procedure for the Elderly*. Windsor: NFER–Nelson.

Shah, S., Vanclay, F., and Cooper, B. (1989) 'Improving the sensitivity of the Barthel Index for Stroke Rehabilitation'. *Journal of Clinical Epidemiology*, **42**, 703–709.

Snaith, R.P and Zigmond, A.S. (1994) *The Hospital Anxiety and Depression Scale*. Windsor: NFER-Nelson.

Tyerman, R.T., Tyerman, A., Howard, P., Hadfield, C. (1986) *Chessington Occupational Therapy Neurological Assessment Battery (COTNAB)*. Nottingham Rehabilitation.

Unsworth, C.A., and Duncombe, D. (2004) *AusTOMs for Occupational Therapy*. Melbourne: La Trobe University.

Webster, C.D., Douglas, K.S., Eaves, D., and Hart, S.D. (1997) *HCR-20: Assessing the Risk for Violence (Version 2)*. Vancouver: Mental Health, Law, and Policy Institute, Simon Fraser University.

Whiting, S., and Lincoln, N. (1980) 'An ADL assessment for stroke patients'. *British Journal of Occupational Therapy*, **43**(2): 44–46.

Chapter 6

Effective Communication for the OT Student

Tracey Polglase and Rachel Treseder

Introduction

This chapter will address a range of communication issues pertinent to professional practice for an occupational therapy student. It will initially consider the different types of communication and communication skills. There will then be a brief overview of communication theory and the link between teamwork and communication. Three examples of good practice for communication in different placement settings will be presented and the key drivers governing professional communication will be tabulated.

Definition

Communication can ultimately be defined as the giving and receiving of information between two or more parties. Although this is seemingly a simplistic definition, communication is a complex process that occurs on many levels.

Types of Communication

Generally communication is either in a verbal or written form. However non-verbal communication also has a huge impact on communication. Baptiste (2010) argues that the importance of non-verbal communication cannot be overestimated. Any form of communication must comply with the stipulations highlighted in College of Occupational Therapists (COT) 2010a and 2007, Health Professions Council (HPC) 2007, 2008 and 2010 and World Federation of Occupational Therapists (WFOT) 2005.

Verbal

Verbal communication involves directly speaking to one or more people. As can be seen in Table 6.1 below verbal communication can be split into informal and formal methods. Some of the examples are in both categories, but the content will indicate which category it belongs in, e.g. a video conference may be used for an in-service training session across a number of sites (informal), or it may be used by the interagency inter-professional team based in different venues for a case conference (formal). Appropriate use of professional terminology is very important. When liaising with colleagues it is important for the student to use professional terminology, whereas when speaking to service users it is important to avoid jargon as this may lead to confusion and alienation.

Table 6.1 Verbal communication

Informal	Telephone conversation
	Video conference
	Discussion with colleagues
Formal	Ward round
	Case conference
	Planning meeting
	Telephone conversation
	Video conference

Non-verbal

Non-verbal communication is a key component of effective communication. Donnelly and Neville (2008, p. 28) argue that:

> In an average face to face communication words make up 7% of a message; tone, tempo and syntax 38% and body language 55%.

This suggests that although words are important how they are presented has greater significance. Non-verbal communication is essentially from the giving and interpreting of facial expression or body language. In some placement settings image/dress code is also a key component, e.g. more casual dress when working with teenagers may impact positively in rapport development as they may interpret those in formal uniforms/suits as threatening. Non-verbal communication can be given intentionally, e.g. active listening to show interest, or unintentionally, e.g. sighing or looking away from the person when they speak will indicate disinterest. Unintentional 'black looks' are also an example of unintentional non-verbal behaviour.

Rapport

The most effective outcomes can be achieved when there is good rapport between the student/therapist and the service user. McKenna (2010) suggests that in order to develop effective rapport with the service user it is essential that the student/therapist's communication is open and honest. Chant et al., (2002) extend this, suggesting that building a therapeutic relationship requires enhanced levels of self awareness.

Written

Written communication can take a number of forms (see Table 6.2) but the communication is via documented evidence. The document may be hand written, e.g. service user notes, or word processed, e.g. letters, reports, etc. As with verbal communication, written communication can also be divided into informal and formal. The style of the written document will depend on its purpose and who the recipient is, e.g. a letter to the GP would be written more formally using professional terminology, whereas a letter to a service user who is well known may be written more informally and using no, or less, professional terminology. As a professional/trainee professional it is important that all documents are accurate, clear and free from spelling and grammatical errors.

Table 6.2 Written communication

Informal	Email
	Fax
	Notes
	Memos
	Telephone messages
Formal	Letters
	Reports
	Service user records
	Email
	Fax

Communication Skills

Much literature has been produced on communication skills and the importance of effective communication skills in healthcare. Brown and Bylund (2008) and Rider et al. (2006) both highlighted in their articles that doctors' effective communication skills have a positive impact on healthcare outcomes. Brown and Bylund's (2008) study goes on to suggest that communication skills are not always optimal but that they can be taught.

Communication skills training can be taught in various ways. Cegala and Broz (2002) undertook a systematic review of 26 intervention studies of communication skills training and concluded that communication skills training is effective in improving the communication skills of doctors, but they also highlighted that in a number of the studies, it was not clear what skills were taught, there were misalignments between skills and the assessment and there was rarely an overarching framework for organising communication skills. Within occupational therapy the majority of assessment of communication skills is undertaken on practice placement. It is therefore imperative that educators are aware of the theory and have a process for accurate assessment.

McCabe and Timmins (2006) suggested that there are a number of core communication skills:

- Active listening
- Questioning
- Body language
- Paralinguistics (tone, pitch, accent, speed)
- Touch
- Information giving
- Establishing rapport
- Empathy.

Marcil (2007) picks one of these, active listening, and argues that it is involved in most communication. Active listening can be conveyed by body language, acknowledging (mirroring) and clarification.

The non-verbal elements of communication have been addressed by Egan (2007). He presented a technique using the acronym 'SOLER' to assist in effective communication by using non-verbal skills positively.

S Sit squarely in relation to the service user/person.
Bodily orientation towards the service user/person.

O Maintain an 'open' posture and do not cross arms or legs. This is non-defensive.

L Lean slightly towards the service user/person. This can be flexible.
Avoid leaning too far forward or too far back.

E Maintain reasonable and comfortable eye contact. Avoid staring or regularly looking away.

R Relax. Avoid fidgeting/becoming distracted. Be comfortable with personal contact.

Egan (2007) and Burnard and Gill (2009) recognise that these guidelines do have a western cultural bias, e.g. some people from Asian cultures would maintain less eye contact naturally than that accepted in Western culture. Students would need to take this into consideration when communicating with people from a non-western culture. Egan (2007) supports a fellow counsellor who argued that with visually impaired individuals eye contact may be less important, but this can be replaced by 'Aim'; aligning head and body to the service user/person in order for them to hear clearly. In this instance **SOLER**, becomes **SOLAR**.

Hobson (2006, p. 102) specifically highlights the importance of environmental influences on communication. She argues that 'an environment with low ambient noise and high ambient lighting (without glare) will optimise communication'. When undertaking occupational therapy assessments it is important for students to consider this, e.g. an initial interview on a busy ward behind a curtain at the bedside is likely to be less effective/successful than one conducted in a private quiet room, without distractions and with comfortable lighting.

Communication Theory

It is important for professionals and students to have an understanding of communication theory and to apply these principles in practice.

Miller and Nicholson (1976) developed the 'Linear Model of Communication'; this is a simple model that has three basic components: sender, message and receiver. The model indicates that the message is relayed from one person to the other in a straight line. In analysing communication it has been found to be a far more complex process than this conveys.

A more comprehensive model, 'The Circular Transactional Model of Communication' Bateson (1979, cited in McCabe and Timmins, 2006), includes the three basic components (sender, message and receiver), but brings in the interpersonal element, which highlights that all communication takes place within a relationship. This model also acknowledges the intrinsic and extrinsic factors that impact on communication. The final additional elements are 'feedback' and 'validation'. Bateson (1979) argues that these are essential for the further development and success of communication. The cyclical dynamic nature of this model indicates the greater complexity of the process.

The Link between Teamwork and Communication

Within the workplace and during academic studies students need to be aware of the importance of effective teamwork. As with communication theory there are also a number of theories guiding team building and team working. Two of the key authors in this respect are Tuckman (1965) for team building and Belbin (2011) for team working.

Tuckman and Jensen (1977) developed the original model to present a five-stage process for team building:

- Forming
- Storming
- Norming
- Performing
- Adjourning/Mourning.

All teams pass though these stages during their development. When there is dysfunction it is evident that the team is stuck at a stage.

Belbin (2011) looked specifically at the roles people undertook in a team. He identified nine key team roles that team members possess in order to function effectively:

- Plant
- Monitor/Evaluator
- Co-ordinator
- Investigator
- Implementer
- Completer/finisher
- Team worker
- Shaper
- Specialist.

If some or any of these elements are missing the team's performance is adversely affected.

Effective team building and teamwork are not possible without effective communication. It is therefore important to consider these two issues in relation to one another.

Examples of Good Practice in Communication Situations for Students

Contributing in multi-disciplinary meetings/case conferences

It is important to remember that when communicating in this type of forum the student is a representative of the OT service and as such should act as a responsible and professional member of that service.

Gathering and sharing information in this type of meeting is often daunting initially, but it is an essential requirement of the role. This anxiety can be reduced by being organised and prepared. COT (2010a Section 5) clearly documents the duties in relation to collaborative working:

- Student to discuss with the educator what to expect and the format of the meeting prior to attending.
- Prior to contributing in the meeting students are often taken as observers so they can familiarise themselves with the protocols.
- Students to make notes prior to the meeting on what they plan to feed back and ask. These can be taken into the meeting and used as a back-up if required. What specifically needs to be presented can be agreed with the educator prior to the meeting.
- Student to be aware that if they are unsure of any details they can ask for clarification from the educator or if no educator present inform the meeting that this is something that they will need to check and feed back later.

- It is important to feed back the key information concisely but including all essential factual information. Beware of subjective information.

Writing an occupational therapy report

Documentation is essential and is stipulated in COT (2010 a & b) and HPC (2007, 2008, 2010).

All reports should be:

Well structured, to include:

- Introduction/type of report
- Service user details, e.g. name address, age, social situation, etc.
- Factual details of the assessment, plan and intervention undertaken
- Summary
- Action plan (if required)
- Contact details of the author
- Date, signature and designation.

Timely:

- Reports should be written within a short period after the conclusion of the assessment/ intervention. Suggested time scale would be no longer than one week. The department may have this stipulated in their 'Standards of Practice'.
- If the intervention is long term, there may be interim reports at specified times.

Professionally written:

- Grammatically correct
- Without spelling errors
- Unambiguous
- Objective and factual rather than subjective
- Using appropriate professional terminology
- Avoiding excessive abbreviations
- Evidencing clinical reasoning.

All documentation, whether it is a written report, an update in the notes or a message taken over the phone, should be written to the same professional standard. If the information is vague or inaccurate there could be serious consequences. Many therapists are 'struck off' the register and unable to work due to poor documentation.

Sample home visit report

Below is a sample Home Visit Report that evidences the standard to which a report should be written:

Name: Mrs Francis Smith   **Date of Birth:** 08/01/1925

Address: 45 Manor Road, XX,XX. AB12 3CD

Tel. Number: (0123) 123456

Next of Kin: Mr John Smith (Husband)

Diagnosis and Presenting Problems

- Mrs Smith was admitted to hospital following a fall five days ago. She had minor injuries: laceration to forehead which was sutured, bruising to right hand and right knee. There were no bony injuries on X-ray.
- She has a long-standing painful right hip and is awaiting an orthopaedic review for total hip replacement. She has limited mobility with a zimmer frame.
- She has a painful left shoulder due to gout and marked osteoarthritic changes.
- There is an ulcer on her right calf which is being dressed daily by the nurses.

Past Medical History

- Osteoarthritis
- Right total knee replacement (2005).
- Ischaemic heart disease and triple bypass (2001)
- Recurrent chest infections
- Asthma.

Social History

Mrs Smith lives with her husband in a 3-bedroomed, privately owned bungalow on a large plot. The village is small, with a post office and shop nearby. They have two daughters, both work full time. One daughter lives locally and the other lives 200 miles away, both are supportive to their parents. Mrs Smith has a private cleaner once a week who also takes Mr Smith shopping once a week. Mrs Smith's husband has memory problems but is able to offer her physical assistance with activities. Prior to hospital admission Mr and Mrs Smith undertook household tasks together. Mr Smith manages to collect the pension from the local post office. Mrs Smith manages all the finances.

Those Present

Mrs Francis Smith (Service User)
Mr John Smith (Husband)
Jane Pool (OT)
Richard Flint (Physio)
Sophie Ray (Social Worker)
Hazel Jones (District Nurse)

Environment

There is a gently sloping drive from the road down to the bungalow. At the front door there are two steps and a handrail on the right to access the property. All rooms lead off a central corridor. There is a large lounge, a dining room, small kitchen, three bedrooms, family bathroom and a separate toilet. The property is spacious and there are no loose rugs on the floor. There is oil fired central heating throughout and an open fire in the lounge. A community alarm system is in place. Mrs Smith has a riser recliner chair in the lounge. There is a frame on each toilet and a seat in the shower.

Service User's Performance

Mobility and Transfers

Mrs Smith was able to walk to the property and around the property using the zimmer frame and close supervision of one person. She required assistance to transfer out of the car and to ascend the steps into the property. She was able to transfer on and off her chair using the raiser/recliner function. Mrs Smith was not able to step into the shower or transfer on/off the shower stool. She required minimal assistance to transfer on and off the toilet using the frames. Mrs Smith needed assistance to transfer into and out of bed. She had difficulty lifting her legs onto the bed and manoeuvring herself in the bed.

Domestic Activities

Mrs Smith was able to make a hot drink and snack in the kitchen as long as all items were placed within easy reach. She used a trolley to transfer items and to take the drink and snack to the dining room. Mrs Smith found this tiring and said she would find making a full meal difficult. The Social Worker provided information on frozen foods.

Personal Activities

Mrs Smith has been assessed washing and dressing on the ward. She can manage to wash and dry some of her top half but has difficulty with lifting her right arm due to the shoulder problems. She requires assistance with washing and drying her bottom half.

Mrs Smith can manage to partially dress herself. She requires assistance with lifting her right arm into blouses and cardigans, but can manage to fasten buttons. She is unable to reach her feet and this impacts on her ability to put on trousers/skirts and shoes and socks. She can pull clothes up if they are put over her feet.

Instrumental Activities

Mr and Mrs Smith undertook household tasks together prior to her admission into hospital. On the visit Mrs Smith was able to wash up the dishes and tidy the bed after she used it for transfers. She would not be able to manage laundry, heavy housework e.g. hoovering or changing the bed.

Summary and Recommendations

Mrs Smith managed some tasks on the home visit, i.e. making a hot drink and snack, but required assistance and supervision to ensure safe transfers and mobility. She also requires assistance with some instrumental activities. The following are recommendations for a safe discharge. *These must be in place prior to discharge:*

1. Social Worker to set up a short term care package for six weeks to assist Mrs Smith with personal care each morning (washing and dressing) and undressing and assisting into bed in the evening. A weekly domestic call is required for laundry, hoovering and changing the bedding.

2. Social Worker to arrange for frozen foods to be delivered five times a week.

3. Social Worker to provide forms for attendance allowance and assist with completing them if required.

4. District Nurse to visit four times a week for wound management.

5. Physiotherapist to arrange for community physiotherapy once a week to provide a rehabilitation programme to improve mobility and transfers.

6. Occupational therapist to advise on falls prevention and the removal of any hazards in the home.

Signature and Designation:

Date:

Recording in Notes

Therapists and students are required to record:

- The aims/goals for the service user
- The intervention undertaken
- The service user's performance and progress/decline
- Any communication with relatives or other professionals/services.

The notes may be electronic or hand written. There are different styles depending on the setting. The student should familiarise him/herself with this early in the placement and follow the protocol of the department.

A good tip is to read the information recorded in the notes and ask yourself whether you could continue the therapy with the service user given the information recorded. If the answer is no, go back and amend the notes. The notes should be comprehensive enough to allow another person to pick up the record and continue the therapy.

Taking a Message

Ensure the following are recorded:

- The person's name and contact details

- The person's professional status or personal status
- Clear details of the message
- Date and time the message was given
- Who took the message
- Details for return call if required, i.e. time, date, contact number, emai,l etc.

Legislation and Policy/Guidance Governing Communication Practice

Tables 6.3 and 6.4 list the key legislation and policy that impacts and drives communication practice.

Table 6.3 Key legislation

Legislation
Access to Health Records Act (1990)
Data Protection Act (1998)
Freedom of Information Act (2000)
Freedom of Information (Scotland) Act (2002)
Mental Capacity Act (2005)
Human Rights Act (Article 8) (1998)
Public Interest Disclosure Act (1998)

Table 6.4 Key policy and guidance

Policy and guidance
Professional Standards for Occupational Therapy Practice (COT, 2007)
Code of Ethics and Professional Conduct (COT, 2010a)
Record Keeping (COT, 2010b)
Mental Capacity Act 2005 Code of Practice (Dept. of Constitutional Affairs, 2007)
Standards of Proficiency: Occupational Therapists (HPC, 2007)
Standards of Conduct, Performance and Ethics (HPC, 2008)
Guidance on Conduct and Ethics for Students (HPC, 2010)
Code of Ethics (WFOT, 2005)

Conclusion

This section highlighted the principles of communication whilst on placement, i.e. what constitutes good and poor communication. Different methods of communication were analysed, e.g. written, verbal, non-verbal, listening, formal and informal. The use of communication skills and the link between positive team working and communication was also evaluated. The importance of communication in the supervision process was highlighted. Key legislation and policy guiding good practice was tabulated at the end of the chapter.

Reflective Questions

1. Consider a team that you have worked in and analyse its effectiveness using Belbin's team roles.

2. Reflect on your own strengths and weaknesses in relation to communication. How might you develop your skills?

References

Baptiste, S. (2010) 'Enabling communication in a person-centred, occupation-focused context' in M. Curtin, M. Molineux and J. Supyk-Mellson. *Occupational Therapy and Physical Dysfunction: Enabling Occupation*. Edinburgh: Elsevier, pp.151–160.

Belbin, M. (2011) *Belbin Team Role Theory*. Available at www.belbin.com (accessed 26/04/12).

Brown, R.F. and Bylund, C.L. (2008) 'Communication skills training: Describing a new conceptual model'. *Academic Medicine*, **83**(1): 37–44.

Burnard, P. and Gill, P. (2009) *Culture, Communication and Nursing*. Harlow: Pearson Education Ltd.

Cegala, D.J. and Broz, S.L. (2002) 'Physician communication skills training: A review of the theoretical backgrounds, objectives and skills'. *Medical Education*, **36**: 1004–1016.

Chant, S., Jenkinson, T., Randle, J., Russell, G. and Webb, C. (2002) 'Communication skills training in healthcare: A review of the literature'. *Nurse Education Today*, **22**: 189–202.

College of Occupational Therapists (2007) *Professional Standards for Occupational Therapy Practice* (2nd edition). London: College of Occupational Therapists.

College of Occupational Therapists (2010a) *Code of Ethics and Professional Conduct*. London: College of Occupational Therapists.

College of Occupational Therapists (2010b) *Record Keeping* (2nd edition). London: College of Occupational Therapists.

Department of Constitutional Affairs (2007) *Mental Capacity Act 2005 Code of Practice*. London: The Stationery Office.

Donnelly, E. and Neville, L. (2008) *Communication and Interpersonal Skills*. Exeter: Reflect Press Ltd.

Egan, G. (2007) *The Skilled Helper. A Problem-Management and Opportunity-Development Approach to Helping*. Belmont: Thomson Brooks/Cole.

Health Professions Council (2007) *Standards of Proficiency: Occupational Therapists*. London: Health Professions Council.

Health Professions Council (2008) *Standards of Conduct, Performance and Ethics*. London: Health Professions Council.

Health Professions Council (2010) *Guidance on Conduct and Ethics for Students*. London: Health Professions Council.

Hobson, S.J.G. (2006) 'Using a client-centred approach with older adults'. In T. Sumsion, *Client-centred Practice in Occupational Therapy*. London: Churchill Livingstone, pp. 91–106.

Marcil, W.M. (2007) *Occupational Therapy: What is it and How does it Work?* New York: Thompson Delmar Learning.

McCabe, C. and Timmins, F. (2006) *Communication Skills for Nursing Practice*. Basingstoke: Palgrave Macmillan.

McKenna (2010) 'Psychosocial support' in M. Curtin, M. Molineux and J. Supyk-Mellson. *Occupational Therapy and Physical Dysfunction: Enabling Occupation*. Edinburgh: Elsevier, pp.151–160.

Miller, G.R. and Nicholson, H.E. (1976) *Communication Inquiry: A Perspective on Process*. Reading: Addison-Wesley.

Rider, E.A., Hinrichs, M.M. and Lown, B.A. (2006) 'A model for communication skills assessment across the undergraduate curriculum'. *Medical Teacher,* **28**(5): 127–134.

Tuckman, B. (1965) 'Developmental sequence in small groups'. *Psychological Bulletin,* **63** (6): 384–399.

Tuckman, B. and Jensen, M. (1977) 'Stages of small group development revisited'. *Groups and Organizational Studies* **2**(4): 419–427.

World Federation of Occupational Therapists (2005) *Code of Ethics*. Forrestfield: WFOT.

Chapter 7

Supervision on Placement

Tracey Polglase and Rachel Treseder

Introduction

This chapter will explore the topic of supervision for the student whilst on placement. In addition to providing a definition, it will consider theory and evidence relating to supervision, and describe different modes of supervision that may be used on placement. It will also provide some suggestions on how to get the most out of supervision during practice placements. As this chapter will focus on supervision on placement, more information on supervision as a qualified therapist can be found in Chapter 9.

Definition

The supervision process is multifaceted and as such a succinct definition is difficult to offer. However its function is to facilitate the development of the student/professional in order to enhance the service offered to the organisation and the service user.

Direct and Indirect Benefits of Supervision

The following table summarises the direct and indirect benefits of supervision.

Table 7.1 Direct and indirect benefits of supervision

Individually focused direct benefits	Service focused indirect benefits
Increase skill development	More effective staff
Increase in knowledge	Highly skilled workforce
Development of clinical reasoning	Practice that is evidence-based
Development of reflective practice	Better service to the service users
Development of professional skills	Improved service outcomes
Evidence for CPD	Meeting the Governance agenda
Positive impact on confidence	

Recommendations for Good Practice in Supervision

- Department to create standards of practice and communicate to all staff
- Supervisors to be provided with training before undertaking the role
- Where possible, supervisor and supervisee to agree to the pairing
- Agree a model to follow
- Record the outcome of each session and both parties sign
- Set action plans with time restrictions and review at each supervision
- Audit the process.

Supervision Theory and Evidence

There is much literature produced on supervision, however it is evident that despite occupational therapists engaging in this process there are likely to be challenges with it. Sweeney et al. (2001 a,b,c) claim that in their study the supervisor and the supervisee felt uncomfortable with the process of supervision.

Evidence suggests that although staff are involved in the process they are ill equipped for it with limited training, poor understanding of the theories and inadequate structures to frame the process. These issues were clearly recorded in Morley's (2007) and Sweeney et al.'s (2001) studies.

It may be useful to use a model of supervision to structure the process. There are a number of models that have been developed; the most commonly used is Proctor (1986). However many of these models are dated, therefore this chapter is presenting a new Process Model of Supervision that can be used by students and practitioners to reflect modern practice. Figure 7.1 indicates this model in diagrammatic form and Table 7.2 presents the functions under each of the three sections. The facilitation role is undertaken by the supervisor to enable the supervisee to progress in professional and therapeutic skill development.

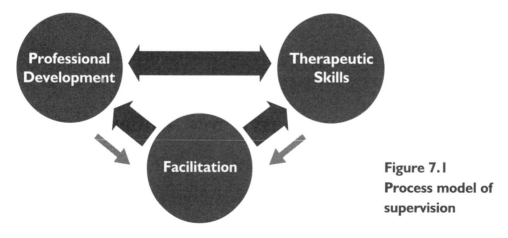

Figure 7.1 Process model of supervision

Table 7.2 Functions within the process model of supervision

Facilitation	Professional Development	Therapeutic Skill Development
Nurturing Challenging Informing Questioning	Communication Reflection Professional Identity Self Awareness Prioritisation & Time Management Research Skills	Therapeutic Skills – i.e. groupwork, environmental adaptation, splinting etc. Problem Solving Process Application of Theory and Evidence-based Practice

The supervisor is responsible for leading the facilitation and the variety of roles indicated in Table 7.2 and these can be used individually or collectively within the supervision session. The supervisee must take responsibility for engaging in the process in order to develop professional and therapeutic skills. The elements are varied and some examples are provided in Table 7.2 although this list is not exhaustive. Although Figure 7.1 indicates that the focus of supervision is on professional and therapeutic skill development of the supervisee, it must be acknowledged that there is a reciprocal arrangement as the supervisor also develops their skills of supervision during the process (professional skill) and through the discussion increase his/her knowledge regarding therapeutic skills (as indicated by the smaller paler arrows).

Types of Supervision Modes of Delivery on Placement

Formal supervision can take the form of different delivery modes depending on the setting, the educator's preference or the number of students placed. The following list indicates the most common modes of delivery.

One to one: The student has one key identified educator who is responsible for managing the placement experience and leads all the supervision sessions. This is the most common and traditional method.

Two to one: The student has two educators with shared placement management and supervision responsibilities. This often happens where there are two educators who work part time or where there is an experienced and an inexperienced educator.

One to two: The educator has two students. This tends to happen where the educator is more experienced. Peer supervision or support is often evidenced in this mode.

Long-arm supervision: Professional supervision is from a designated educator or academic tutor who is not based at the placement setting. This is usually seen on a role emerging placement, see Chapter 8 for more details

Peer/group supervision: Students are on placement in pairs or groups and/or have the opportunity to meet whilst on placement. Peer or group supervision is an invaluable mechanism of support.

Pyramid supervision: This combines long-arm supervision from an educator alongside peer supervision, where experienced final level students offer some supervision to the less experienced students.

How to make the most of supervision on placement

Supervision is likely to take two forms;

- Informal
- Formal.

COT (2008) suggests that supervision in both a formal and an informal context is essential to the placement experience and student learning.

Informal supervision is unstructured, occurs continually throughout the placement and will provide the student with opportunities to reflect on practice through discussion with the educator and other team members. This is a valuable learning opportunity and gives the student the chance to undertake 'reflection in action'.

Informal supervision and feedback throughout a placement has an equal value to the placement experience and to guide learning. Students perceive constructive and positive feedback as a facilitator of learning and promoter of self confidence (Löfmark and Wikblad, 2001). Therefore, timely discussion and regular feedback on a day-to-day basis serve to benefit the student and their development of knowledge and skills.

Formal supervision is structured and should be offered at least once a week for a minimum of one hour during the practice placement. This offers the opportunity to review the progress to date, the learning objectives and set an action plan for the forthcoming week/s. This should be documented so there is a clear record of the topics discussed during the meeting and an action plan to guide the remaining time of the placement. Documentation serves to bring transparency, clarity and explicit guidance for both the educator and student to draw upon in the placement learning. It also minimises misunderstanding over progress and goals to be achieved. To make the most out of the supervision available, the student and the educator need to prepare for the supervision by actively reflecting on the learning to date. Use of a supervision model may be utilised to structure the session.

Supervision can be an invaluable part of the learning experience and offers opportunities to reflect on practice and gain support and guidance from the practice educator so that the student can develop both personally and professionally (Clouder and Sellars, 2004).

Craik (2009) suggests the essence of supervision is to bring clarity of purpose agreed between the student and educator and a willingness to engage in open discussion. There is a need for trust, respect, rapport and a proactive approach to the process, where all parties need to come prepared, allow sufficient time and record the outcomes. Alsop and Ryan, (1996) argue that supervisory relationships thrive on good communication and interpersonal skills.

At times supervision can be an uncomfortable process for the supervisee and the supervisor. The giving and receiving of constructive criticism needs to be done professionally and sensitively.

Preparation for Supervision

In order to get the most from supervision it is important to prepare for it. Below is a list of things that a student or therapist can do in preparation for their supervision sessions:

- Undertake written reflections on critical incidents throughout the week and bring them to the supervision to discuss what has been learnt from them. A range of reflective models could be used and these could also be evaluated in relation to the process of reflection.

- Work as a reflective practitioner throughout the week.

- Attend a journal club and feed back key learning from the articles discussed. Indicate how this knowledge can inform practice.

- Bring a list of the things to be discussed and the priority, just in case there is not time to cover everything.

- Review the previous supervision report and check that all the activities planned have been achieved. If they have not, consider why this has not happened.

- Review the plans achieved and the ones still outstanding. Consider the priority for the ones outstanding.

- Evaluate progress to date and the things to be achieved. Take ownership of these and be proactive in the learning process.

- Always ensure there is a written record of all supervision sessions and review this throughout the week.

Conclusion

This chapter has highlighted the importance of a good supervision process for both the student and the educator in order to enhance the placement experience. It has identified some of the theory and evidence supporting the need for supervision, and the variety of modes of delivery that can be used. Practical suggestions have been discussed in light of this theory, to encourage both the student and educator to make the most of the supervision process. Further discussion of transferring these skills to practice as a qualified therapist can be found in Chapter 9.

Reflective Questions

1. Consider your experience of supervision on placement. What modes of delivery were used? How prepared were you? How effective was the supervision?

2. What knowledge and skills relating to supervision can you transfer to your future placements/practice?

References

Alsop, A. and Ryan, S. (1996) *Making the Most of Fieldwork Education: A Practical Approach*. Cheltenham: Nelson Thornes Ltd.

Clouder, L., and Sellars, J. (2004) 'Reflective practice and clinical supervision: An interprofessional perspective'. *Journal of Advanced Nursing*, **46**(3): 262–269.

College of Occupational Therapists (2008) *College of Occupational Therapists Pre-registration Education Standards* (3rd ed). London: College of Occupational Therapists.

Craik, C. (2009) 'Practice education: skills for students and educators'. In E. Duncan (ed.) (2009) *Skills for Practice in Occupational Therapy*. Edinburgh: Churchill Livingstone, pp. 323–335.

Löfmark, A. and Wikblad, K. (2001) 'Facilitating and obstructing factors for development of learning in clinical practice: a student perspective'. *Journal of Advanced Nursing*, **34**(1): 43–50.

Morley, M. (2007) 'Developing a preceptorship programme for newly qualified occupational therapist: Action research'. *British Journal of Occupational Therapy*, **70**(8): 330–338.

Proctor, B. (1986) 'Supervision: A co-operative exercise in accountability'. In M. Marken and M. Payne (eds) *Enabling and Ensuring: Supervision in Practice*. Leicester: National Youth Bureau, Council for Education and Training in Youth and Community Work, pp. 21–34.

Sweeney, G., Webley, P. and Treacher, A. (2001a) 'Supervision in occupational therapy, part 1: The supervisor's anxieties'. *British Journal of Occupational Therapy*, **64**(7): 337–345.

Sweeney, G., Webley, P. and Treacher, A. (2001b) 'Supervision in occupational therapy, part 2: The supervisee's dilemma'. *British Journal of Occupational Therapy*, **64**(8): 380–386.

Sweeney, G., Webley, P. and Treacher, A. (2001c) 'Supervision in occupational therapy, part 3: Accommodating the supervisor and the supervisee'. *British Journal of Occupational Therapy*, **64**(9): 426–431.

Part 3

Looking Ahead

Chapter 8
The Future of the Profession

Rachel Treseder

Introduction

This chapter will discuss the role of practice education in supporting the development of the profession. In addition to reflecting the current climate of employment opportunities in the statutory sector within the UK, issues in relation to the profession's increasing awareness of its philosophical roots and the need to expand its scope of practice will be explored. Specific areas of innovative practice will be discussed. Case studies for each of these areas will illustrate pertinent issues.

Innovative Practice

1. Role emerging placements.
2. Inter-agency placements.
3. Management placements.
4. Overseas placements.

There is a growing awareness that occupational therapy is a complex intervention (Creek, 2003). The complexity arises from the concept of occupation itself and the interplay of the individual and their environment and the multitude of intrinsic and extrinsic influences that impact on health and well-being.

As occupational therapy is being redefined and re-conceptualised in the twenty-first century, there is evidence of evolving debate in the academic and political arena (Watson and Swartz, 2004; Pollard et al., 2008, Creek and Lawson-Porter 2007). General societal issues such as governmental policy and legislation, changing social contexts and demographics will all influence the future of the profession. Similarly, advances in theoretical knowledge and research will contribute to the development of the profession. The evolving discipline of occupational science and related concepts such as occupational deprivation, occupational injustice and apartheid all form part of the evolutionary process of the profession.

However, amidst the debate and discussion from an intellectual perspective, there is an inevitable question arising: what impact is this actually having, and will have, on practice? This chapter will aim to present the 'bottom-up' approach that practice education and students can have in promoting occupational therapy in new and innovative areas of practice through role emerging placements. It will illustrate through the use of real-life case studies, how students can learn about the value of occupation and the dual purpose of these placements, in applying the developing theoretical concepts in practice. There will also be an exploration of the evolution of roles in the statutory sector and how practice education relates to these.

Role Emerging Placements

A role emerging placement is a practice placement occurring at a site where there is not an established occupational therapy role (College of Occupational Therapists, 2006). The student, or potentially students, will work within the organisation alongside the current service that is provided, and identify a potential occupational therapy role. This may be with a specific individual, or group of individuals. This can often take the form of a project with an occupational focus that mirrors the occupational therapy process.

Role emerging placements were first introduced as a concept in the 1970s (Overton et al., 2009) but have developed significantly in the last decade. The rationale for this has been attributed both to the shortage of placements in the traditional areas of practice, and the changing health and social care arena, necessitating a widening scope of experience required for students. Some universities have now adopted a whole cohort model which requires all students to undertake a role emerging placement at the same stage in their training (Thew et al., 2008).

The World Federation of Occupational Therapists (Hocking and Ness, 2002) has acknowledged the importance of students experiencing a depth and breadth of experience in their placements. The College of Occupational Therapists (2006) have responded to the development in role emerging placements by publishing guidelines for students, higher education providers and service providers in the effective implementation of these placements.

Supervision models (see Chapter 7 for more details)

Models of supervision on role emerging placements take several forms. One of the most common is the tripartite arrangement between student, on-site supervisor and long arm supervisor (see Figure 8.1 below).

On-site supervisor

The student will receive ongoing support from the on-site supervisor who will not be an occupational therapist, but provide the support and supervision required for management/organisational issues.

They will be the first point of contact for the student whilst on placement, and contribute to the assessment process throughout.

Long-arm supervisor

Whilst on any placement the student must have some form of supervision from a registered occupational therapist even though they don't necessarily need to be on site (Hocking and Ness, 2002; College of Occupational Therapists, 2007). This supervision within a role emerging placement may be a tutor from the student's higher education institution, or a therapist in an area that reflects the organisation where the placement is taking place. Although the student inevitably has less day-to-day contact with their supervisor, there is regular supervision time planned, usually once a week, or once a fortnight. There may be opportunities for the supervisor to observe the student in practice, although the main focus of the supervisory relationship is on reflective practice and clinical reasoning. The long-arm supervisor will also be involved in the assessment process throughout the placement.

Student

In role emerging placements students are frequently placed in pairs or groups. This provides an opportunity for peer supervision. Students will often work on projects together and the support that this provides is vital when there may be limited understanding of occupational therapy within the organisation.

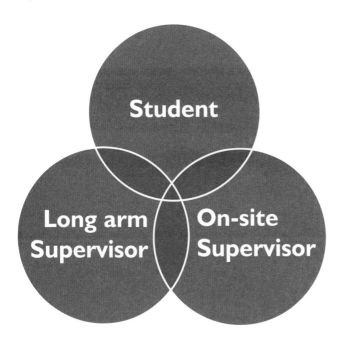

Figure 8.1 Tripartite arrangements for supervision in role emerging placement

Some examples of organisations where a role emerging placement may take place are homeless hostels, young person's charities, nursing/residential homes, learning disability workshops, prisons, hospices or schools. The main criterion for the compatibility of organisations in hosting occupational therapy students is that there is an element of, or potential for an occupational focus within the service, and scope for developing this within the placement timescale. The case studies below aim to illustrate this further.

Table 8.1 Case study 1: Young person's charity

Background
Two occupational therapy students have been allocated to a role emerging placement for their critical evaluation placement. The placement is 12 weeks long, in a young person's charity within an inner city. The charity aims to work with young people between the ages of 13 and 25 who have disengaged with statutory services such as mainstream education and employment. This is mainly achieved through a programme of activities and projects that aim to develop life-skills through creative means. It is a voluntary service so all the young people are there through choice. The charity is funded through grants and private donations. There is a staff team of a service manager, threee development tutors that work directly with the young people, two outreach workers that collaborate with outside organisations, a fundraiser, an administrator and a number of volunteers.

Supervision and assessment of the students
The students are being supervised by one of the development tutors on-site, and by one of their university OT tutors on a weekly basis. They also provide peer supervision for each other. They used their learning contract throughout their placement to identify their specific learning needs for the placement, and this is monitored by both the on-site supervisor and long-arm supervisor.

The OT Process: Assessment
The OT students are invited to join the development tutors and a group of six young people who have been recently referred to the service, on an access course. This is a three-day residential course in the local countryside where the young people will be camping and undertaking a number of outdoor activities as part of their introduction to the programme. Every young person who is referred to this service will go on an access course as part of the assessment process. This provides opportunity for therapeutic relationships to be established and young people to commit to other projects that are offered.

During the course the OT students participate in all the activities that are led by the development tutor, including kayaking, gorge walking, and coasteering. Through these activities and their interaction with the young people, they identify that three of the young people have very low self-esteem and confidence in their ability to perform, but respond significantly to positive reinforcement and encouragement. Through observation of the young people at mealtimes it also becomes apparent that all of the young people have very limited knowledge of healthy eating and food hygiene.

The OT students develop an assessment form based on the Model of Human Occupation (Kielhofner, 2008) and complete it for all six young people based on their observations at the access course. Although they do not formally interview any of the young people, they are able to gather a substantial amount of information from their informal interactions and observations of daily activities throughout the three days.

Planning

From the information gathered on their assessment forms the OT students are able to identify a number of strengths and needs for each of the young people. They then develop short term aims and objectives for each young person which enables them to maintain a client-centred approach as they plan their intervention session.

Intervention

The OT students decide to run an animation project, which addresses the issue of food hygiene. This will involve the creation of animated characters to resemble specific bacteria, which then are used to illustrate the importance of hygiene when preparing food. Alongside this they also decide to run a healthy eating project, which involves the practical preparation of healthy meals, which the young people will plan, shop, prepare and eat together once a week.

The project is run over six weeks and engages all six of the young people. An educational approach is adopted as the young people learn about food hygiene in a creative, non-threatening way. The client-centred approach adopted also allows each of the young people to develop skills in particular areas through the graded process of the project. These include 'hard skills' such as reading and writing skills, maths skills, camera work, shopping, cooking, budgeting and 'soft skills' such as concentration, communication and working within a team. The occupational focus of the project allows the development of these skills in a non-directive way. The occupational therapy students learn how to manage group dynamics, and provide opportunities for the development of individual skills identified at the assessment stage.

Evaluation

At the culmination of the project the students and young people organise an event to present the animation that they have created at the local arts centre. A number of people are invited including parents, friends, staff and supporters of the charity. A 'healthy' buffet is prepared by the young people for the presentation, which includes the food that they have learnt how to prepare during the project.

Observation of the young people during this event allows the students the opportunity to re-visit their original assessment information and record any progress they have made in specific areas. Specifically, a number of the young people have grown in confidence in their newly acquired skills. They re-visit their short-term goals with the OT students and identify longer term goals, which include signing up to a cooking course in college, continuing to prepare healthy food for themselves at home within a budget, and working towards qualifications to achieve a place on an animation degree course.

Reflection on the placement

The OT students completed a number of reflections through the process of the placement, which were used in supervision. There were several periods of significant learning due to frequent periods of feeling 'overwhelmed' and a little lost by the limited direction provided by educators which they had been used to in the past. This had been viewed as an opportunity to learn rather than a threat and the core principles and philosophy were re-visited by the students in order to identify what the role of an OT may look like in this setting.

Their final reflection demonstrated a significant development in learning transferable skills such as professional identity, confidence, communication, the value and adaptation of occupation as a therapeutic intervention.

Inter-agency placements

An inter-agency placement involves the student being based between two different, but connected organisations for their placement. The occupational therapist within one organisation would take the responsibility for the student, but will collaborate with an additional service that may be linked such as within the voluntary or private sector (Fisher and Savin-Baden, 2002). The student will spend time in both organisations and use the opportunity to develop collaborative links and integrated working between services. This type of innovative placement contributes to the College of Occupational Therapists' agenda for increased collaborative working (College of Occupational Therapists, 2002).

Students will receive the majority of their supervision from the occupational therapist although they may also require an element of supervision from a member of staff from the participating organisation who may not be an occupational therapist. This follows a similar pattern to the supervision model in role emerging placements, except that there will be more contact working alongside the registered occupational therapist.

Table 8.2 Case study 2: Elderly day hospital and social services
(with thanks to Sue Baker)

Background
A student has been allocated to an inter-agency placement between health and social services. The student will spend three half-days in an NHS Day Hospital for elderly people and one day in Social Services. There was an occupational therapist in each setting and all parties met prior to the placement to agree the following: Objectives of placement   Learning opportunities across the two sites   Number of days at each site   Supervision and assessment structure   Selection of student – i.e. previous experience, access to a car etc.   Ethical considerations – i.e. the student offered patients a quick seamless service across the two sites, thus avoiding the waiting list   Communication – i.e. between the two educators and across the two sites

Supervision and assessment of the students
The lead supervisor was the occupational therapist working in the Day Hospital as this was where the majority of the time was spent. Informal supervision was regular and ongoing between both supervisors and the student. Formal supervision sessions were held on a weekly basis and there was regular communication between all three parties on a regular basis. The student was assessed by the occupational therapist in their respective settings and at the end of the placement they decided on the assessment outcome and completed the report together.

Day Hospital
The student attended the daily multidisciplinary meeting in the Day Hospital where all patients for that day were discussed. Within this meeting new referrals were allocated and the student was given a caseload that he was responsible for. Each patient referred was initially interviewed in the Day Hospital and further assessments including a home visit were arranged if required. The service user attended the Day Hospital for an initial 12 weeks during which the student undertook the whole OT process of assessment, planning, intervention and evaluation.

Social Services

The student was either allocated service users from the waiting list in Social Services or retrieved the referrals he had made in his role within the Day Hospital earlier in the week. Under the guidance of the occupational therapist he worked within the remit of social services with his caseload to provide suitable equipment to aid independence.

Reflection on the placement

Benefits to practice education team and organisations:

Increased awareness and communication across two departments

Increased awareness of documentation needs of two departments

Provided seamless service between two areas

Reduction of duplication of work Health/Social Service OTs

Compatible with national and COTs guidelines on collaborative working (COT 2002)

Changed outlook and practice

Benefits for student:

Experience across two services

Access to both supervisors and their experiences

Access to both organisations' resources for service users

Service user focused

Improved communication skills both verbal and written

Enjoyable and challenging

Benefits for service users:

Seamless service between Health and Social Services

One contact throughout OT intervention

Challenges of the placement:

Challenging for the student to only be in social services setting one day a week

Student having to learn two different documentation systems

Practice education team/educators needed to ensure the standards expected of the student were equitable to other students at his level.

Management Placements

A further example of innovation in practice education is management placements. These placements provide opportunities to work alongside current occupational therapy managers with the specific purpose of developing management skills and understanding the role of an occupational therapy manager in more depth.

The vision for occupational therapy education is that students develop competence in the areas of knowledge, skill and professionalism (COT, 2009, p. 7) in order to move the profession towards changes needed in the current climate. In addition to providing an invaluable experience for the student, these placements also provide opportunities for managers to maintain their contact with students and ensure their supervision skills continue to be developed.

The College of Occupational Therapists (2009) have identified a common statement of the profession's expected graduate competencies and there are particular competencies relating to management skills that are expected of new graduates (see Table 8.3)

Table 8.3 Expected graduate management skills in the leadership and promotion of occupational therapy

The occupational therapy graduate is able to:
Determine and prioritise occupational therapy services.
Understand and apply the principles of leadership and management to occupational therapy services, including the establishment of occupational therapy protocols.
Engage in a continuous process of evaluation and improvement of the quality of occupational therapy provision, involve users of services where appropriate and communicate results to others.
Take a proactive role in the development, improvement and promotion of occupational therapy.
Proactively seek out and influence policies and legislation in health and social care locally, nationally and internationally that impact on occupational therapy service.

(College of Occupational Therapists, 2009, p. 12)

There is little evidence to suggest how management skills are developed in undergraduate occupational therapy students, although there is clearly an emphasis placed on the need that they should be (Adamson et al., 2001; COT, 2009; Moyers, 2007).

Management placements are an example of how students can focus on developing management skills that will be expected on qualification. The following case study provides a real life example of how this was achieved.

Table 8.4 Case study 3 Management placement

Background
A student has been allocated to a placement with a manager of occupational therapy services for mental health. The occupational therapy manager, a member of the practice education team and the student met prior to the placement to discuss the following:
Focus of the placement – i.e. choice of specific project to ensure learning outcomes were achievable. How the learning outcomes for the occupational therapy process/therapeutic skills could be interpreted in this placement.
Ethical considerations – i.e. what was appropriate for the student to be involved in due to issues of confidentiality and sensitive information.
Supervision and assessment of student
The supervision structure was traditional in that the occupational therapy manager provided weekly formal supervision on a one-to-one basis. Similarly the occupational therapy manager assessed the student through her learning contract and her performance throughout the placement.
Some roles undertaken during the placement:
Attended trust wide meetings as a representative of the occupational therapy department.
Developed audit criteria for evaluating the mental health element of the occupational therapy service.
Involved in the writing of the report for the service review, which was linked to the service critique assignment for university.
Attended occupational therapy departmental staff meetings.
Developed standards for supervision and undertook responsibility for disseminating these to the occupational therapy staff.
Contributed to service development, i.e. setting up a new vocational rehabilitation group with occupational therapists on the ward.
Contributed to a presentation of the placement at a national conference.
Reflections
The student reflected that the placement enabled her to:
Gain a better understanding of Clinical Governance in terms of service development. Improve professional communication skills.

Learn about the importance of using discretion and maintaining confidentiality.

Improve self confidence when communicating to other professionals and senior staff.

Gain an understanding of the problems faced by managers on a daily basis.

Gain a better understanding of legislation governing service provision and the pressures exerted on managers.

Understand the importance of communication and difficulties that can be experienced through poor communication.

The educator reflected that having a student:

Provided further evidence for Continuing Professional Development and maintaining skills in supervising students.

Was an excellent learning experience.

Enabled occupational therapy to be promoted at management level.

Was useful to have a reciprocal exchange and discussion of relevant literature, issues and evidence-based practice.

Developed confidence from valuable feedback on performance from the student.

International Placements

There are now 53 countries that are full members and 10 associate member countries of the World Federation of Occupational Therapists (WFOT, 2010). The profession is developing globally as well as nationally, and with this a broadening scope of opportunity for OT students to gain a depth of experience from different cultures.

There are a variety of methods that students may use to gain experience from another country. Very often students choose to undertake their final elective placement in another country as this placement is usually not assessed, and students are more responsible for organising this placement themselves. However, this section will concentrate on two other main forms of international placement: the ERASMUS scheme and undertaking an assessed placement in an overseas country.

The ERASMUS Scheme *(with thanks to Gareth Morgan)*

ERASMUS stands for European Community Action Schemes for the Mobility of University Students. ERASMUS is the EU's flagship education and training programme enabling 200 000 students to study and work abroad each year. In addition, it funds co-operation between higher education institutions across Europe. An overriding aim of the programme is to help create a 'European Higher Education Area'.

ERASMUS became part of the EU's Lifelong Learning Programme in 2007 and covered new areas such as student placements in enterprises (transferred from the Leonardo da Vinci Programme), university staff training and teaching for business staff. The programme should further expand the educational opportunities it offers in the coming years, with a target of 3 million ERASMUS students by 2012.

How ERASMUS Works

Universities, which participate in ERASMUS activities, must have an ERASMUS University Charter. The Charter aims to guarantee the quality of the programme by setting certain fundamental principles. The European Commission is responsible for the overall programme implementation; its Directorate-General for Education and Culture coordinates the different activities. So-called 'decentralised actions' that promote individual mobility are run by national agencies in the 33 participating countries. The National agency in the United Kingdom is the ERASMUS UK arm of the British Council. For further information see http://ec.europa.eu/education/erasmus/doc890_en.htm (accessed 26/04/12).

Clinical exposure

Within professional practice it is an aspiration that occupational therapy students are exposed to new experiences, which challenge their assumptions, and practice during their placement. It also gives them the opportunity to reflect on new challenges and action new interventions within perhaps a more challenging cultural and social environment. This is accompanied by the opportunity to live and work in a foreign country, which naturally embraces other opportunities and challenges student experience. Students are enabled to travel for a minimum of three and a maximum of twelve months to encourage immersion in the experience. They benefit from a mandatory, non-means tested grant from the scheme, which helps to subsidise the visit. It does not, however, cover the total cost of the experience. As an exchange programme the ideal scenario exists if an incoming student is replaced by an outgoing one.

Table 8.5 Case study 4: ERASMUS scheme (with thanks to Alexander Smith)

Background
This case study will describe the experiences of an occupational therapy (OT) student. participating in the ERASMUS exchange programme in Gothenburg, Sweden. The exchange consisted of a 12-week critical evaluation placement, in a specialist neuro-rehabilitation hospital. Service users were aged between 18 and 65, diagnoses were varied, yet remained within the overarching label of neurology.
Supervision and assessment of the student
The supervision consisted of on-site supervision from the student's educator and fortnightly supervision from a member of the host university's academic staff. Additionally there was a half-way visit from the student's home university tutor, to evaluate the student's learning contract and progression with their learning needs.

Assessment

Within this setting assessment was to be carried out within the first week of arrival at the hospital. A wide array of assessments were available, which enabled broad assessment of occupational difficulties. In turn this enabled the therapist to focus on specific areas of difficulties whilst a member of the multi-disciplinary team (MDT) conducted a Functional Independence Measure (FIM) (1999) baseline assessment (Dittimar and Granger, 1997).

Planning

The planning process of this setting, involved every member of the MDT in addition to the clients and their families. In concurrence with the client-centred modality of practice, planning meetings were designed to empower the service user. This was achieved by each health professional justifying and clarifying to the service user the interventions which they believed would best assist the service user in achieving their goals.

Intervention

In relation to intervention a strong client-centred and MDT approach was adopted. The OT was required to accommodate the interests of service users in relation to the interventions offered, whilst upholding the principle that all service users were required to receive 45 minutes of OT per day. In regards to the MDT, many therapeutic interventions were conducted as joint sessions with a myriad of MDT members.

The types of interventions afforded to the service users were extremely varied. However an evidence-based approach was taken, when utilising any intervention. Interventions ranged from the recognisable OT interventions such as activities of daily living (ADL) type interventions, to gardening groups and a breakfast group at the start of the week. Whilst planned group activities were an important aspect of rehabilitation, the majority of the service users' rehabilitation was on a one-to-one basis. This allowed for increased flexibility for the service user and demanded increased flexibility of the therapist on the service user's behalf. In the daily one-to-one sessions, service users were free to ask beforehand for specific activities that were enjoyable to them. In consequence, and in keeping with an evidence-based approach, tasks were analysed prior to commencement, to ascertain therapeutic gain. As a result, the types of intervention or therapeutic activity were diverse and included: shopping practice at a local supermarket, visiting a large inner city shopping complex to practice walking in crowds and to overcome the social anxiety of changes in posture and gait; to more simplistic therapeutic activities such as the re-potting of house plants or creating tie dye cloth.

In addition to the service user-led interventions, it was also necessary to implement structured intervention programmes related to the service users needs upon discharge such as transfers, mobility, cooking and other ADLs. Furthermore there was a strong academic presence in the hospital, which resulted in a number of research studies based around OT interventions, such as virtual reality training.

Evaluation

As with other aspects of the OT process, evaluation was based around the goals agreed by the service user and the MDT in the planning process. Professionals would evaluate a service user's progress benchmarked against an admissions FIM score. This process was discursive and involved all professionals in equitable manner. Moreover service users were able to voice their opinion on their progress regularly and individual professionals constantly evaluated the efficacy of their interventions

Reflection on the placement

Whilst on placement the student completed a number of reflections. These reflections related to issues such as cultural isolation and becoming enamoured with Swedish modality of practice. The student found in Sweden an appreciation for client-centred practice with a greater MDT input which they felt was lacking in their experiences of the UK.

An Assessed Placement Overseas

In order for a student to complete an assessed placement overseas, the country they are travelling to must be a full member of the World Federation of Occupational Therapists (see www.wfot.org for a list of these countries). There are a number of practical issues that must be addressed if a student is considering a placement abroad:

- Insurance and Visa – the student must hold indemnity insurance which is provided by COT. The student will have this insurance when they register as a student in the UK. The student must also have travel insurance – some universities will provide this free of charge. NB This will only cover for the period of the placement and not any additional travelling that the student may decide to undertake. Some receiving countries will require the student to have a working visa in order to undertake their placement. It is the responsibility of the student to ascertain the requirements.

- Information about the receiving organisation – it is important that the student is fully aware of the resources available (i.e. staffing and environment) and that these fulfil requirements for them to achieve their learning outcomes.

- Requirements of the student's home university – the practice education team are obliged to ensure that students are sent to a placement that fulfils health and safety requirements. It may be a requirement for the university to sign a contract with the host organisation.

- Supervision and assessment arrangements – expectations are that these will follow the guidelines set by the university.

- Expenses – it is the student's responsibility to fund the expenses attached to this placement (e.g. travel, accommodation and any other related expenses) with the exception of the ERASMUS scheme as discussed earlier.

Table 8.6 Case study 5: Overseas placement (with thanks to Gill Drury and Kat Ball)

Background
Two occupational therapy students organised a 14-week evaluation placement in a secondary school in Cape Town, South Africa. The students were based at the school and supervised by occupational therapists employed there. They were working in a team, which included teachers, counsellors and psychologists. The students also had the opportunity to work at a drug rehabilitation centre and in community outreach sites.
Supervision
Having occupational therapists already employed in this setting meant that supervision and information were readily available; this is obviously different to many other international and role-emerging settings. Peer support was very valuable and all elements of supervision were a significant part of the placement experience.
Occupational Therapy Planning and Intervention
During the three month placement the students helped to plan and facilitate classroom sessions to teach 'Life Orientation' (similar to personal, social and health education in the UK). The occupational therapy process was focused on a prevention model rather than an intervention model of practice. This was a very different approach to those seen in occupational therapy settings around the UK. It took several weeks to build an understanding of the desired outcomes for the occupational therapists in this setting.
In the centre the OT students planned and facilitated a weekly arts and crafts group for the residents.
Managerial staff from the Life Orientation department were also involved in the management of the drug rehabilitation centre for adolescents.
Finally, in community outreach work, the students introduced occupational therapy programmes into a pre-school and adult disability home in a socio-economically deprived area near to the school.
Opportunities and Challenges
This placement gave the students a huge range of challenging and exciting learning experiences with different opportunities for autonomy and creative practice than in UK settings.

Some of the challenges about having a placement overseas were in practicalities such as: financial restraints and time planning. Other challenges revolved around learning and understanding the occupational therapy aims and interventions within this setting.

Also, learning and negotiating the cultural differences that exist in occupational therapy practice situations was a major consideration, e.g. building cross-cultural rapport and understanding the occupational therapy role.

Conclusion

This chapter has explored some of the new and innovative areas that occupational therapists are developing into, and how students and practice education have a key role in supporting this development. It has identified some of the opportunities and challenges that are presented for students undertaking placements in these settings, and the importance of rigorous support and supervision in this process.

Reflective Questions

1. What do you think you would personally find most challenging about an innovative placement opportunity?
2. What skills do you think it would help you to develop?
3. In which innovative settings do you think occupational therapists could use their skills?

References

Adamson, B.J., Cant, R.V. and Hummell, J. (2001) 'What managerial skills do newly graduated occupational therapists need? A view from their managers'. *British Journal of Occupational Therapy*, **64**(4): 184–192.

College of Occupational Therapists (2002) *From Interface to Integration: A Strategy for Modernising Occupational Therapy Services in Local Health and Social Care Communities*. London: College of Occupational Therapists.

College of Occupational Therapists (2006) *Developing the Occupational Therapy Profession: Providing New Work-Based Learning Opportunities for Students*. London: College of Occupational Therapists.

College of Occupational Therapist (2007) *Professional Standards for Occupational Therapy Practice* (2nd edition). London: College of Occupational Therapists.

College of Occupational Therapists (2009) *Curriculum Guidance for Pre-Registration Education*. London: College of Occupational Therapists.

Creek, J. (2003) *Occupational Therapy Defined as a Complex Intervention*. London: College of Occupational Therapists.

Creek, J. and Lawson-Porter, A. (2007) *Contemporary Issues in Occupational Therapy: Reasoning and Reflection*. Chichester: John Wiley & Sons.

Dittimar, S.S. and Granger, G.E. (1997) *Functional Assessment and Outcome Measures for the Rehabilitation Health Professional*. Maryland: Aspen, pp. 7–9.

Fisher, A. and Savin-Baden, M. (2002) 'Modernising fieldwork, part 2: Realising the new agenda'. *British Journal of Occupational Therapy*, 65(6): 275–282.

Hocking, C. and Ness, N.E. (2002) *Revised Minimum Standards for the Education of Occupational Therapists*. Perth: World Federation of Occupational Therapists.

Kielhofner, G. (2008) *Model of Occupation: Theory and Application*. 4th edition. Baltimore: Lippincott Williams & Wilkins.

Moyers P.A. (2007) 'A legacy of leadership: Achieving our centennial vision'. *American Journal of Occupational Therapy*, 61(6): 622–628.

Overton, A., Clark, M., and Thomas, Y. (2009) 'A review of non-traditional occupational therapy practice placement education: A focus on role-emerging and project placements'. *British Journal of Occupational Therapy*, 72(7): 294–301.

Pollard, N., Sakellariou, D., and Kronenberg, F. (2008) *A Political Practice of Occupational Therapy*. London: Churchill Livingstone Elsevier.

Thew, M., Hargreaves, A. and Cronin-Davis, J. (2008) 'An evaluation of a role-emerging practice placement model for a full cohort of occupational therapy students'. *British Journal of Occupational Therapy*, 71(8): 348–353.

Watson, R. and Swartz, L. (2004) *Transformation through Occupation*. London: Whurr Publishers Ltd.

World Federation of Occupational Therapists (2010) *Member Countries of WFOT*. Available at www.wfot.org (accessed 26/04/12).

Chapter 9
Becoming a Newly Qualified Occupational Therapist

Tracey Polglase

Introduction

The ultimate aim for any occupational therapy student is to successfully pass the course and to be able to work as an occupational therapist. This chapter aims to provide some insight into how practice education can contribute towards becoming a qualified occupational therapist through developing transferable skills that increase a student's employability. It will also present a framework of the processes required in order to secure a post, advise on mandatory requirements and continuing professional development (CPD) activities and provide information on preceptorship and other support mechanisms, all of which are important for the student to know.

Registration with the Health and Care Professions Council

The Health and Care Professions Council (HCPC), formerly Health Professions Council, was set up under the Health Professions Order 2001. It replaced the Council for Professions Supplementary to Medicine (CPSM) and has wider powers. The HCPC currently regulates 16 professions and aims to protect the public by setting standards that the professionals need to meet. The HCPC is responsible for:

- Approving education programmes
- Maintaining a register of approved professionals who can use the 'protected titles'
- Setting standards for professionals to achieve
- Monitoring CPD
- Considering complaints about a registrant from members of the public and taking appropriate action.

In order to work in the UK an Occupational Therapist needs to be registered with the HCPC.

How to Register

New graduates can register once they have confirmation from their university that they have satisfactorily completed the course of study. The university will send a list of all new graduates to HCPC. The student then needs to complete the application form. This is accessed from the website (www.hcpc-uk.org).

Tips for completing the form:

- Ensure a black pen is used
- Read the Guidelines for Completing the Form
- Follow the instructions carefully
- Complete all sections
- Use the checklist at the front of the form to ensure all forms are completed and documents enclosed in the envelope when posting
- Only send certified copies of documents requested. There is a list of the documents accepted and who can certify them
- Do not use paperclips or staples
- Enclose payment mandate rather than cheque, this means that you will never miss a payment and accidentally be removed from the register. It is a difficult process getting back on the register and you cannot work as an OT during this time
- The Health Declaration Form needs to be signed by the applicant. Don't forget to get the Character Reference Form completed. The person completing this form must have known the applicant for at least three years
- Don't forget to sign the application form!

In the busy period (July–August) the form can take up to a month to process. Once it has been processed the professional's name will appear on the register and a letter with certificate will be sent to the individual. It is only at this point that employment can commence. If the application form and/ or documents are incorrect the form will be returned for re-submission. This will cause a delay in registration and ability to work.

Registrants must re-register every two years. This involves completing a self declaration form. Two per cent of those on the register will be required to provide evidence of their CPD activities and how this has impacted upon their practice since the last registration.

Securing a Post
Looking for a post
When to look

Most graduates qualify in the summer, however some courses have purposely changed their course completion date to correspond to another key time when posts suitable for newly qualified staff become available. Posts suitable for graduates are often advertised in February/March. There is not a right or wrong time to look for a post. Some students will feel they are unable to focus on preparation for a job when they are in the final six months of their degree, which is a stressful period. Others feel more content when they know they have a post secured.

Where to Look

- The *British Journal of Occupational Therapy* and *Occupational Therapy News*. Most UK occupational therapy posts are advertised in the professional journal. These are available to all therapists and students who are members of the British Association of Occupational Therapist as a hard copy and online (www.cot.org.uk).
- All NHS posts are also advertised on the local intranet services and the NHS jobs website (England and Wales – www.jobs.nhs.uk, Scotland – www.jobs.scot.nhs.uk, Northern Ireland – www.n-i.nhs.uk). Councils often have monthly publications where local authority posts are advertised. Also look at the local council's website jobs section.
- Local press advertise some posts.
- Charity publications, e.g. *Big Issue*.

Although the majority of graduates seek employment in occupational therapy specific posts, there is a growing trend towards graduates recognising that their skills developed from placement, and wider skills can be used in other posts; this is particularly evident in the third sector. In order to prepare for this most universities now offer students the opportunity to experience a placement in a role emerging setting.

Finally, although posts all need to be advertised, sometimes this is only done internally. Making contact with local departments and keeping them informed of your continued interest in posts may just remind them to notify you when a post becomes available.

What level of post to apply for?

As will be discussed later in the chapter the transition from graduate to newly qualified therapist is often challenging. Additional support is offered to those joining the profession at the graduate entry position, through the preceptorship process. There is no professional restriction on what level of post can be applied for, however the personal specification may indicate previous experience or length of time since qualification. Despite this there are still some graduates who secure posts higher than entry level, e.g. Band 6. It is recommended that new graduates choose posts that are at entry level. This allows for development of a solid foundation of personal and professional knowledge and skills to support the specialist skill acquisition later in the career. A weak foundation can lead to problems later.

Choosing the Right Post

The next decision revolves around choosing the right post. There are a number of considerations.

Where?

In order to focus the search, it is useful to have an idea of geographical location. Most newly qualified therapists seek employment in the UK initially. As long as the therapist is registered with HCPC they can work in any OT post. There are different rules and regulations for overseas employment. Each country will provide the specific requirements in order to apply and work there, e.g. visa, entry exams, etc.

The next decision is which sector to work in. Most occupational therapists work within the health sector (NHS). The next most common sector is social care (local authority). A growing field is the third sector (charities and voluntary organisations). Posts in the third sector may not be occupational therapy posts, but require occupational therapy skills. Even if occupational therapists do not work in occupational therapy posts as long as they can indicate how they have maintained their professional skills they can continue to be registered with the HCPC. There are also a number of occupational therapists that work in the private sector, (national private organisation or small companies). Newly qualified therapists tend to start work in the health or social care sectors, while more experienced staff work in the third sector and in private practice. Choice of sector may depend on availability of positions, but placement experience can also influence a choice of first positions. Skills developed on placement can be largely transferable across sectors so do not limit job applications according to placement experience. Be creative in demonstrating how skills can be transferred across sectors and settings.

Type of post

Most posts for newly qualified staff are full time in nature (approximately 37.5 hours), however it is possible to secure part time posts, but these tend to be in static positions.

Secure or locum

All secure posts are either permanent or temporary/fixed term. A permanent post means that there is no set end date. The post is available as long as the therapist wants to remain there. If the organisation wishes to withdraw the post they will need to pay redundancy according to the terms and conditions of the organisation. A temporary/fixed term post is for a specific period (e.g. two years). After that period the post will cease and the therapist will need to look for another post. There will be no redundancy pay.

In the current economic climate employers are moving away from permanent posts and towards temporary/fixed term posts. N.B. securing loans, mortgages, etc. is more difficult when your employment is on a temporary/fixed term contract.

The other type of post available is a locum post. Therapists sign up with an agency and when suitable employment opportunities arise the agency links the therapist with the organisation offering the post. The post may be as short as one week or for several months. There are advantages and disadvantages to this type of employment. Some people like the flexibility of this type of working; they can choose when they work, who they work for and leave if they do not like it. Another advantage is that the pay is significantly higher than in a secure post. The disadvantages are the uncertainty of how long the post is available for, there may also be no vacancies in a particular area, the experience may not suit the therapist and the terms and conditions may not be as favourable as in non locum posts.

Rotation or static posts

Posts for newly qualified staff can be rotation or static. A high proportion of posts are offered on a rotation basis. This basically means that the therapist spends a set time in a specific role (e.g. six months rheumatology), then moves to another setting within the organisation or link organisation (e.g. six months community mental health). This process continues until the therapist secures a static post within the organisation, moves or gains promotion to a more senior post. Most staff will stay in a rotation post for 18 months to two years. A rotation post allows the novice therapist to develop skills in a number of fields and therefore assists them in deciding where they wish to specialise. Equally it may also inform them of areas that they do not want to specialise in. The other obvious benefit is that it develops a broader range of skills, thereby creating a more holistic therapist.

Static posts also have their benefits. Some therapists are very sure of the area they want to work and specialise in. If this is the case and a static post becomes available in that field, the therapist would be able to develop skills from an early stage in their career, without working in a range of settings that they are less interested in. This may also suit some therapists who need to work in a specific location, without the need to move.

Completing the Application Form

It cannot be stressed how important it is to get this aspect right. This is likely to be the first contact between the applicant and the short listing panel. A poorly completed application form will often be rejected irrespective of the content. In the current climate there may be 50 or more applicants for a post, therefore the application form needs to stand out positively from the rest. The application form may be in electronic form or hard copy.

Tips for Completing Application Forms

- Read the Guidelines for Completing the Form
- Follow the instructions carefully
- Complete all sections fully
- The Personal Statement section is the most important. Ensure this is well detailed and focused on applying your knowledge and skills to this post
- Don't forget to sign the application form!
- Enclose a CV if the application allows it. If not take one to the interview and give it to the panel
- Ensure the application form is completed and sent to arrive before the closing date

- If sending by post send by recorded delivery
- If sending electronically ask for a confirmation of delivery.

References

Referees should be chosen who can clearly and honestly comment on either the applicant's professional skills or personal attributes. Most application forms ask for two referees. The first one should be the current employer (if applicable) or if newly qualified, the Programme Manager of the course just completed. The second referee can be someone who knows the applicant professionally or personally. They will need to indicate in what capacity they are known. Relatives cannot act as referees.

Applicants should always ask the referees if they would be willing to give a reference prior to putting them on the form. Once the applicant knows that they have an interview they should then inform the referee. References can be tailored to the job being applied for, therefore by keeping the referee informed the reference is likely to be more structured and meaningful to the post.

Applying for Posts

The Curriculum Vitae (CV)

Focus the CV to the post you are applying for – 'one size does not fit all'. They also need to be regularly updated. There are different formats for CVs, but the general rule is that there are certain elements that are essential:

- Personal Details
- Personal Statement
- Education History/Qualifications
- Placement History (if newly qualified)
- Work History (Paid and Voluntary)
- Relevant Courses.

Preparation for the Interview

Applicant to:

- Undertake an informal visit prior to the interview. (This will give him/her the opportunity to meet the staff, ask questions and check out the department. The interview is about deciding if the applicant wants the post as well as the panel deciding if they want the applicant.)

- Think about questions (factual and hypothetical) that may be asked and practice answering them. Consider skills that have been developed on placement that can be transferred to the specific setting that is being applied for.

- Ask experienced staff what sort of questions may be asked.

The Interview

Applicant to:

- Always arrive early. (Allow plenty of time just in case of unexpected delays on the journey.)
- Always present the answer to the panel member that asked the question. Try to give as full an answer as possible. There is no problem with thinking about the answer for a short time before giving it. This may allow articulation of the information in a more logical format.
- Ensure the presentation (if required) looks professional. This often assesses a lot more than the content, i.e. organisation, research skills, communication skills, articulation of information, etc.
- Always bring the professional portfolio to an interview. (It may not be asked for, but it shows a well organised applicant.)
- Ask some questions at the end of the interview. (It is acceptable to have a prepared list of questions that can be used.)
- Confirm what will happen following the interview.
- Thank the panel for the interview.

Post Interview

Applicant to:

- If unsuccessful ask for feedback on how to improve in the future.
- Be accessible via the contact details given.
- Undertake any requests e.g. providing documents such as CRB checks, attend induction.

Starting Work

Preceptorship

Although preceptorship is fairly new for therapists in the UK, it has been used in nursing since the early 1990s. Preceptorship was introduced with Agenda for Change (DoH, 2005). The process is now a stipulation of all NHS contracts. It was put in place for newly qualified staff to assist them in the transition from graduate to competent professional. Much literature has highlighted the challenges faced by new graduates and evidence suggests that specific support during this period can assist the novice therapist to transfer and develop their skills, knowledge, professional identity and confidence.

It takes at least one year to complete the preceptorship process. Although legislation stipulates the requirement for a preceptorship system it does not indicate the structure, implementation or evaluation requirements. Many places have therefore adopted an informal process with limited measurement. In contrast to this, Morley (2009) undertook a study evaluating a formalised preceptorship programme for occupational therapists. Preceptees were required to undertake specific tasks at set periods. The preceptor offered constructive feedback, support and advice throughout the period as well as questioning around clinical reasoning. At the 6-month and 12-month stage the preceptee was measured against the Knowledge and Skills Framework (KSF) outline (DoH, 2004) and if considered to have met the agreed targets received a pay rise. From the findings of this study she offered a new definition for preceptorship for occupational therapists:

> Preceptorship is a structured development process, including observed practice and feedback against agreed standards, to support newly qualified practitioners to build their professional identity and competence in order to facilitate their successful adaptation into the workplace.
>
> (Morley, 2009a, p. 388)

Morley (2009b) has recently published the second edition of the *Preceptorship Handbook for Occupational Therapists*. This addition also includes the COT Standards of Practice, KSF Profiles and the HPC standards for CPD. Further information is also now available in DoH (2010) which sets out preceptorship guidelines for organisations. This document has been produced for nurses, midwives and allied health professions.

Quick et al. (2007) suggest a partnership agreement between academic and practice to support new graduates through the transition process to competent professional. It could be argued that this would assist in bridging the theory–practice divide and has the potential for therapists to maintain their academic development following qualification. They can be supported by academic staff to transfer skills in seeking evidence to support practice, and publishing material gained through research activities. This would increase the evidence-based literature available, which is often limited.

Activities within the preceptorship process are undertaken uni-professionally to develop the knowledge, skills, professional identity and confidence of a newly qualified graduate. In order to develop this further it is proposed that the activities that are undertaken in the safety of the one-to-one process could be extended for more experienced staff into an interprofessional context. This would assist the individual to define their role, understand other professionals' roles and jointly agree how the roles complement each other for the benefit of the service user. Interprofessional standards could be set and practice measured against these. An interprofessional system would also be beneficial for those staff working in small departments where they may be the only occupational therapist in the team.

Supervision

Supervision is one component of the preceptorship process but should continue throughout a therapist's career.

COT (2010, p. 30, 5.4.5) Code of Conduct stipulates:

> You should be supported in your practice and development through regular professional supervision within an agreed structure or model. Sole practitioners should seek out professional support and advice for themselves.

The supervision process is multifaceted and as such a succinct definition is difficult to offer. Its function is to facilitate the development of the professional, in order to enhance the service offered to the organisation and the service user.

There is much literature produced on supervision, however it is evident that despite occupational therapists engaging in this process there are problems with it. Sweeney et al. (2001 a,b,c) claim that in their study the supervisor and the supervisee felt uncomfortable with the process.

Evidence suggests that although staff are involved in the process they are ill equipped for it with limited training, poor understanding of the theories and inadequate structures to frame the process. These issues were clearly recorded in Morley's (2007) and Sweeney et al.'s (2001) studies.

It may be useful to use a model of supervision to structure the process. There are a number of models that have been developed (see Chapter 7 for detail on the Process Model of Supervision). Again it is important for therapists to transfer skills learnt from placement in the supervision process.

Coaching

Over the last decade there has been increasing awareness in the UK of coaching, in both personal and professional development arenas. Coaching aims to develop potential and enhance work performance through one-to-one facilitation and challenging guidance (O'Donovan, 2006)).

Driscoll and O'Donovan (2007) argue that there are elements of coaching that can be used in supervision, particularly with senior staff, where the process may be more egalitarian, analytical and less 'problem orientated'. They term this 'Developmental Coaching'. They go on to say that clinical supervision with a more individual and performance related focus is more suitable for novice staff. Despite the differences they suggest the TGROW Model (Downey, 1999 p.29, cited in Driscoll and O'Donovan, 2007) can be used as a framework within the supervision process. The supervisee chooses the topic, the supervisor controls the structure. The supervisee is expected to prepare information prior to the session and send to the supervisor. The supervisor asks questions in relation to each aspect to focus the session.

Other Support Mechanisms

Peer support groups

A number of organisations have peer support groups for staff. These are often run by the group and activities are agreed by the group. They can be group specific, e.g. Band 5 support group, special interest specific, e.g. palliative care support group, or professional development specific, e.g. journal club.

Professional body

In addition to being registered with the HCPC, all occupational therapists, students and support staff have the option of being a member of the British Association of Occupational Therapists. This is the professional body and will provide a range of information and services. BAOT membership forms can be downloaded from www.cot.org.uk.

Membership will entitle the member to have:

- The *British Journal of Occupational Therapy* and *Occupational Therapy News* monthly
- Professional Indemnity Insurance and Unison membership
- Legal guidance and advice
- Professional advice
- Access to the COT library
- Access to professional publications
- Reduced fees for events and publications
- Join committees and specialists sections
- Voting rights
- County and Regional Groups
- Funding for activities, e.g. education, research and CPD activities
- Income Tax Relief on BAOT subscriptions
- International links (COTEC, WFOT).

Continuing Professional Development (CPD)

Activities and portfolio

The CPD portfolio should start to be developed from the outset of their education as an occupational therapist. The HPC (2009) document gives advice on CPD and provides a list of activities that are considered as suitable evidence under CPD. A range of these should be used and evidenced within a professional portfolio. There are various templates that can be used to record CPD. The COT has information on their website www.cot.org.uk and also an interactive database http://ilod.cot.org.uk (Interactive Learning Opportunities Database iLOD) that includes information on formal learning opportunities, career planning and CPD tools. Remember to use placement experiences to reflect transferable skills and knowledge gained, such as the SWOT analysis discussed in Chapter 4. These are important skills that are important to record as part of the CPD process.

TRAMM Model

A new model for CPD developed by occupational therapists is the TRAMM model (Morris et al., 2011). See Figure 9.1. This was developed to reflect the five standards of CPD for HPC (HPC 2009). There are five stations that the individual needs to pass through and record the outcomes from, but there is no specified direction.

Tell

Formulation of learning needs and dissemination of learning outcomes. It is important to plan professional development and to share the knowledge and skills attained. This may happen in supervision, in-service training, publications, etc.

Record

Keeping a record of CPD activity and change of practice as a result of it is required by the HPC. Reflections on practice can be used in this section. The portfolio may be called every two years and has implications for re-registration. The TRAMM Tracker (see below) can be used for this.

Activity

Those things undertaken which facilitate CPD, e.g. attending conferences, being a member of a journal club, shadowing other staff, reading relevant publications, etc.

Monitor

CPD needs to be monitored. There are several ways to do this, e.g. within supervision and through reflection. Mentorship may also be used for this process, particularly with inexperienced staff.

Measure

Setting specific, individualised goals. These may be set at appraisals or during supervision. Performance against them can then be measured at specific agreed intervals.

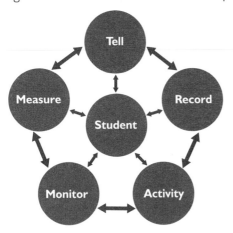

Figure 9.1
TRAMM model (Morris et al., 2011)

Table 9.1 Suggestions for activities that fit into the TRAMM model
(these are not exhaustive and people may choose their own)

T: Tell	
Informal/formal discussions	Journal club
Supervision	Annual appraisals/individual performance Review (IPR)/professional development review (PDR)
Peer supervision	
Disseminating information	Presentations
Facilitating training sessions	Case studies

R: Record	
Current evidence-based practice	Annual appraisals/IPR/PDR
Publications	Portfolio
Service evaluation	Induction material
Reflection – verbal/written	Information leaflets
Learning contracts	Curriculum vitae
CPD record sheet	Audit

A: Activities	
Mandatory and specialist training	Project work
Further education	Member of specialist section/interest group
Learning from colleagues	Involvement in professional body
Shadowing/secondments/rotation	Accreditation and revalidation
Lecturing/teaching	External examining
Reading journals	Research
Attending conferences/courses	
Attending/facilitating workshops	
Reflection	

M: Monitor	
Formal/informal mentorship	Being managed
Supervision – staff/students	Performance indicators
Establishing development plans	Formative assessment
Peer reviews	Competences
M: Measure	
Specific individualised goals	Applied knowledge
Informal education opportunities	Audit
Performance indicators	Outcome measures
Standards of proficiency	Letters of commendation
Skill acquisition and improvement	Research

There is also a TRAMM Tracker, an adaptable electronic or manual tool to record and measure individual learning outcomes against the HCPC's standards. Further information on the model and tracker is available at: orca.cf.ac.uk/18418/1/HEARLE_Final_Draft_AI.pdf (Accessed 26/04/12).

Re-registration

Two per cent of those on the register will be required to provide evidence of their CPD activities and how this has impacted upon their practice since the last registration. This is reviewed and if considered satisfactory, they are re-registered.

Conclusion

This chapter has attempted to direct the reader through the processes and procedures in searching for and securing a position and the support mechanisms available once in post. Finally it has presented information on continuing professional development and a model that can be used for this.

Reflective Questions

1. How might you approach supervision to get the most out of it?
2. Using one of the suggested models analyse how application of this has impacted upon your depth of learning.
3. What are the key things you have learnt from this chapter that you will carry forward to assist you in successfully securing a new job?

References

College of Occupational Therapists (2010) *Code of Ethics and Professional Conduct.* London: College of Occupational Therapists.

Department of Health (2004) *The Knowledge and Skills Framework and the Development Review Process. Final version.* London: The Stationery Office.

Department of Health (2005) *Agenda for Change Terms and Conditions Handbook.* London: The Stationery Office.

Department of Health (2010) *Preceptorship Framework for Newly Registered Nurses, Midwives and Allied Health Professionals.* London: The Stationery Office.

Driscoll, J. and O'Donovan, G. (2007) 'Exploring the potential for professional coaching for the growth of clinical supervision in practice.' In J. Driscoll (ed.) *Practising Clinical Supervision: A Reflective Approach for Healthcare Professionals* (2nd edn). Edinburgh: Balliere Tindall Elsevier, pp. 119–140.

Health Professions Council (2009) *Your Guide to our Standards for Continuing Professional Development.* London: Health Professions Council.

O'Donovan, G. (2006) *A Definition of Life Coaching.* Available at www.noble-manhatten.com (accessed 26/04/12).

Morley, M. (2007) 'Developing a preceptorship programme for newly qualified occupational therapists: Action research'. *British Journal of Occupational Therapy,* **70**(8): 330–338.

Morley, M. (2009a) 'An evaluation of a preceptorship programme for newly qualified occupational therapist'. *British Journal of Occupational Therapy,* **72**(9): 384–392.

Morley, M. (2009b) *Preceptorship Handbook for Occupational Therapists* (2nd edn). London: College of Occupational Therapists.

Morris, R., Salmon, T., Lawson, S., Leadbitter, A., Morris, M., and Mandizha-Walker, M. (2011) 'Creativity through appreciative inquiry.' *Occupational Therapy News,* **19**(6): 26–27.

Quick, L., Forsyth, K. and Melton, J. (2007) 'From graduate to reflective practice scholar'. *British Journal of Occupational Therapy,* **70**(11): 471–474.

Sweeney, G., Webley, P. and Treacher, A. (2001a) 'Supervision in occupational therapy, part 1: The supervisor's anxieties'. *British Journal of Occupational Therapy,* **64**(7): 337–345.

Sweeney, G., Webley, P. and Treacher, A. (2001b) 'Supervision in occupational therapy, part 2: The supervisee's dilemma'. *British Journal of Occupational Therapy,* **64**(8): 380–386.

Sweeney, G., Webley, P. and Treacher, A. (2001c) 'Supervision in occupational therapy, part 3: Accommodating the supervisor and the supervisee'. *British Journal of Occupational Therapy,* **64**(9): 426–431.

Chapter 10

Conclusion

Tracey Polglase and Rachel Treseder

This chapter will summarise the key points raised in the book.

Introduction

This book was developed to address the needs of students, newly qualified therapists, educators and academic tutors.

Main Body

Chapter 1: What is Practice Education?

This aimed to provide the reader with a clear overview of what practice education is and how it is incorporated into the curriculum, thereby contextualising practice education within the overall education experience. Potential areas where practice education can occur were also presented.

Chapter 2: Theoretical Principles

This chapter was split into two parts; Part 1 presented the development of occupational therapy and practice education from its inception through to current practice. Part 2 reviewed learning theory with a particular focus on adult learning.

Chapter 3: Preparation of Students for Placement

This chapter is specifically valuable for students and academic tutors as it indicates what should be included in planning and preparing students to go out on placement.

Chapter 4: The Learning Experience on Placement

This chapter indicates the role and responsibilities of the student and the educator in the education experience. The concept of a collaborative learning approach is presented together with the tools that are used to facilitate this. Assessment and evaluation processes and tools are also explored.

Chapter 5: The Occupational Therapy Problem Solving Process on Placement

This is the largest chapter and so is divided into four sections:

- Assessment knowledge and skills
- Planning knowledge and skills
- Intervention knowledge and skills
- Evaluation knowledge and skills

These four sections replicate the problem solving process. Within the Assessment, Intervention and Evaluation Sections case studies have been used to indicate application of tools/media to practice.

Chapter 6: Effective Communication for the OT Student

The Communication chapter presented the different types of communication and a brief overview of communication skills and communication theory. Tips on good practice for communication in a variety of situations were presented. There was also an indicator of the legislative and policy drivers that influence communication. Communication is considered to be an essential element of practice that underpins all stages of the therapeutic process.

Chapter 7: Supervision on Placement

This chapter identified the importance of supervision on placement and presented some of the theory and evidence on the process of supervision. In acknowledging some of the difficulties and challenges in the supervision process it also presented some advice and guidance on how to make the most of supervision during placement, both for the educator and the student.

Chapter 8: The Future of the Profession

This chapter focuses on some innovations in practice placement and how these are preparing students to be the future graduates of the profession. The profession is evolving both in its own right and in response to economic, political and sociological influences. It is the duty of the higher educational institutions to prepare the future workforce to meet these demands. Exposure to innovative placement experiences is one way this is achieved.

Chapter 9: Becoming a Newly Qualified Occupational Therapist

This chapter introduces the reader to some professional requirements, e.g. registration with the Health and Care Professions Council and the process required to achieve this. There is also a step-by-step outline of choosing a post and the application process. Suggested support mechanisms once the therapist starts work are discussed together with the importance of continuing professional development (CPD). A new tool to support this process is presented.

It is hoped that the contents of these chapters will both inform and inspire (at times!) the reader.

Glossary

Allied Health Profession (AHP): A profession that forms part of the multi-disciplinary team and is affiliated to healthcare but outside of the remit of medical staff. May be from a variety of backgrounds.

APPLE Accreditation: A method of validating practice educators in their assessment of occupational therapy students. The qualification is approved by the College of Occupational Therapists and contributes to providing parity across universities and practice education settings in the training of educators. It is not currently mandatory.

Assessment: The gathering of information at the initial stage of the occupational therapy process in order to inform the planning and intervention of services. This baseline of information can then be used at the evaluation stage of the occupational therapy process in order to measure the effectiveness of the intervention.

Audit: Audit is a process of monitoring performance using specific criteria to measure against. There are a range of tools that can be used for this purpose in order to meet the specific needs. Audit is often a cyclical process whereby specific performance is measured, reviewed, modified and measured again.

Benchmarking: A process that uses a number of organisations in a collaborative arrangement in order to improve quality of service. The organisations involved measure their own performance against each other to seek out best practice. Specific targets are stipulated in relation to performance, efficiency and effectiveness.

British Association of Occupational Therapists (BAOT): The professional body for occupational therapy in the UK.

Care Programme Approach (CPA): A whole process inter-professional approach that is predominantly used in mental health for the planning of care and therapy. There is one set of paperwork that records the assessments undertaken, their results and the plan of action across professional and agency boundaries.

Clinical Reasoning: The professional justification given for any aspect of the therapeutic process undertaken with a service user.

Collaborative Working: The practise of joint working and sharing of information in the therapeutic process for the benefit of the service user and to avoid duplication.

College of Occupational Therapists (COT): A wholly owned subsidiary of BAOT which operates as a registered charity. The College sets the professional and educational standards for the occupational therapy profession and represents the profession at the national and international levels.

Continuing Professional Development (CPD): A requirement stipulated by the Health and Care Professions Council that all healthcare professionals continue their learning and professional development throughout their career. Evidence of this must be kept in a CPD portfolio which is an individual responsibility to maintain.

COT Standards of Practice: Minimum requirements to guide practice for occupational therapy staff. The standards are underpinned by legislation and regulatory and monitoring bodies.

Critical Analysis: Consideration and evaluation of the claims made by the authors whilst judging the credibility of the findings and the relevance to the subject matter.

Curriculum Vitae (CV): A document that records personal and professional qualifications, achievements and accolades.

ERASMUS (European Community Action Schemes for the Mobility of University Students): The European Union's education and training programme enabling students to study and work abroad each year and facilitating co-operation between higher education institutions across Europe.

Evaluation: 'The process of obtaining, interpreting and appraising information (about occupational performance) in order to prioritise problems and needs, to plan and modify interventions and to judge the worth of interventions' (Creek 2010, p. 25)

Evidence-based Practice: Use of credible sources to inform, guide and support the therapeutic process.

Exam Board Ratification: A quality assurance process by external examiners that ensures parity of marking and moderation within the university and maintenance of comparable standards between universities.

Frames of Reference: The conceptual framework on which practice is based.

Holistic practice: Consideration of the whole person within the context of their environment.

Health and Care Professions Council (HCPC), formerly Health Professions Council (HPC): The HCPC is a regulatory body that currently regulates 16 professions and aims to protect the public by setting standards that the professionals need to meet. The Health Professions Council (HPC) was set up under the Health Professions Order 2001.

Innovative placements: The use of new and emerging settings for students to experience the practical element of the programme.

Inter-agency: Two or more different organisations working together – this can be within one organisation or across different organisations (inter-sectoral).

Inter-professional: More than one professional working collaboratively for a common purpose.

Inter-professional education: 'when two or more professions learn with, from and about each other to improve collaboration and the quality of care' (CAIPE 2002).

Intervention: The stage of the occupational therapy process that follows assessment and planning and involves putting the 'plan into action' (Creek 2003).

Intra-professional: Two or more professionals from the same discipline but different organisations working together.

Journal Club: A meeting of colleagues to discuss and share the findings of journal articles on a specific topic.

Knowledge and Skills Framework (KSF): The NHS Knowledge and Skills Framework (the NHS KSF) defines and describes the knowledge and skills which NHS staff need to apply in their work in order to deliver quality services. It provides a single, consistent, comprehensive and explicit framework on which to base review and development for all staff (DOH 2004, p. 1).

Learning Contract: Can be defined as an agreement between a learner and an educator that specifies in detail:

- Learning objectives
- The resources and strategies required to accomplish the objective
- The evidence required to demonstrate the objectives have been accomplished and
- The specific criteria for evaluation/validation.

Long-arm Supervision: Within this model, an educator who is not based directly with the student provides regular formal profession specific supervision. It relies on clinical reasoning and discussion as a supervision tool.

Multi-disciplinary team: A team that is made up of a range of disciplines that work towards a common goal.

Non-standardised Assessment: Assessments that are often designed by individual occupational therapy departments to assess service users but have not been through the rigorous process of testing for reliability and validity.

Occupation: Any activity that occupies one's time to include self care, productivity or leisure activities.

Occupational Analysis: The examination of an individual's participation in an activity that considers both intrinsic and extrinsic factors in its investigation.

Occupational Deprivation: When an individual has a deficit of occupational choice because of social, political, cultural, economic or environmental influences and thus experiences a sense of exclusion.

Occupational Engagement: When an individual is fully immersed and part of an activity.

Occupationally Focused Objectives: Actions with an occupational focus that are specific, graded and measurable, written for the service user to guide them to reach an aim/goal.

Outcome Measures: a standardised instrument used to establish whether a therapeutic outcome has been met.

Planning: The second stage of the problem solving process where aims/goals and objectives are set to inform intervention.

Practice Education: This is the practical element when students undertake their learning in an area of service provision.

Practice Educator: A professional qualified occupational therapist, who has undertaken an accredited course of study to assess students on placement within the workplace.

Reflection: A psychological construct that is closely related to a range of other internal mental (cognitive) processes such as thinking, reasoning, considering and deliberating.

Reflective Journal: A diary used to record critical incidents, therapeutic practice and thought processes to aid and evidence professional development.

Reflective Models: Frameworks to structure the reflective process.

Reflexivity: The impact of a person's values, beliefs, acquaintances and interests on his or her research or work activity

Role Emerging Placement: A practice placement occurring at a site where there is not an established occupational therapy role (College of Occupational Therapists 2006).

Self Directed Study: Students undertaking study independently of direct tutor involvement.

Service User: A recipient of service. Can also be called patient, client or customer depending on the setting.

Single Assessment Process: Professionals from health and social care in England working together collaboratively to assess and provide care to service users.

Standardised Assessment: Assessments that have been rigorously tested under research conditions to guarantee reliable and valid results.

Supervision: A communication process between the supervisor (educator) and the supervisee (student) in order to facilitate the development of professional and therapeutic skills.

Teamwork: Colleagues working together collaboratively for the benefit of the service user or the effective achievement of a task.

Third Sector: Organisations that are funded from charitable sources.

Unified Assessment Process: Professionals from health and social care in Wales working together collaborative to assess and provide care to service users.

World Federation of Occupational Therapists (WFOT): The official representative of occupational therapy and occupational therapists worldwide.

References

Centre for the Advancement of Interprofessional Education (CAIPE) (2002) *Defining IPE*. Available at www.caipe.org.uk/resources (accessed 18/02/12).

DOH (2004) *The NHS Knowledge and Skills Framework (NHS KSF) and the Development Review Process*. London: Crown.

Index